Emergency Survival Skills: Vital Tactics for Survival

Ewen .P Farley

All rights reserved.

Copyright © 2024 Ewen .P Farley

*Emergency Survival Skills: Vital Tactics for Survival :
Master essential skills for surviving unexpected emergencies*

Funny helpful tips:

Rotate between different time periods; literature from various eras offers diverse insights and cultural understanding.

Stay committed to regular sleep patterns; consistency in rest improves energy and focus.

<u>Life advices:</u>

In the meadow of dreams, chase your aspirations with unwavering belief.

Engage with books that promote holistic health; they offer insights into physical, mental, and spiritual well-being.

Introduction

This book serves as a comprehensive and essential guide for individuals seeking to acquire the knowledge and skills required to perform basic life-saving techniques. This manual is designed to equip readers with the step-by-step instructions and fundamental principles necessary to provide life support in various emergency situations.

The manual begins with a focus on adult basic life support (BLS). It covers the fundamentals of BLS, emphasizing the critical importance of prompt and effective intervention in cases of cardiac arrest or life-threatening emergencies. Readers learn about the primary components of BLS, including chest compressions, rescue breaths, and the use of automated external defibrillators (AEDs).

Airway management is a crucial aspect of BLS, and the manual dedicates a section to this vital skill. Proper airway management ensures that a patient's airway remains open and unobstructed, allowing for effective ventilation and oxygenation. Readers are provided with guidelines and techniques for maintaining clear airways in adult patients.

Automated external defibrillators (AEDs) have become increasingly important in saving lives during cardiac arrest situations. The manual includes detailed information on how to use an AED, covering the steps required to operate this life-saving device. Readers gain a thorough understanding of when and how to apply AED shocks to restore normal heart rhythms.

The manual provides step-by-step instructions for performing single-rescuer adult BLS, which is essential for individuals who may find themselves in situations where immediate assistance is required. Readers learn the sequence of actions to follow, from checking for responsiveness to delivering chest compressions and rescue breaths.

In cases where two rescuers are available, the manual also offers guidance on performing 2-rescuer adult BLS. This section outlines the roles and responsibilities of both rescuers to ensure effective and coordinated efforts in delivering life support.

Pediatric basic life support is addressed comprehensively in the manual, recognizing the differences in caring for children and infants. Readers are guided through the fundamentals of pediatric BLS, emphasizing the importance of age-appropriate techniques and interventions.

The manual also covers airway management and AED use in pediatric and infant BLS scenarios, ensuring that readers are well-prepared to respond to emergencies involving younger patients.

Choking incidents are addressed with detailed instructions on how to provide relief to adults, children, and infants. Readers learn the techniques for dislodging obstructing objects and restoring normal breathing in choking victims.

The manual also includes alternate topics, such as the management of opioid-induced emergencies, reflecting the evolving nature of emergency medicine and the need for responders to adapt to new challenges.

Team synchrony is emphasized throughout the manual, recognizing that effective communication and coordination among rescuers are essential for successful outcomes in emergency situations. Readers are encouraged to work together seamlessly to provide the best possible care to patients in need.

In summary, this book is a comprehensive and indispensable resource for individuals seeking to acquire the knowledge and skills necessary for responding to life-threatening emergencies. It covers a wide range of topics related to adult, pediatric, and infant BLS, airway management, AED use, and choking relief. This manual equips readers with the tools and information they need to make a difference in critical situations and potentially save lives.

Contents

ADULT BASIC LIFE SUPPORT 1
    FUNDAMENTALS 1
    AIRWAY MANAGEMENT 10
    AUTOMATED EXTERNAL DEFIBRILLATOR 18
    PERFORMING SINGLE-RESCUER ADULTBASIC LIFE SUPPORT 23
    PERFORMING 2-RESCUER ADULT BASIC LIFESUPPORT 28

PEDIATRIC BASIC LIFE SUPPORT 31
    FUNDAMENTALS 32
    AIRWAY MANAGEMENT 42
    AUTOMATED EXTERNAL DEFIBRILLATOR 50
    PERFORMING SINGLE-RESCUER PEDIATRICBASIC LIFE SUPPORT 55
    PERFORMING 2-RESCUER PEDIATRIC BASICLIFE SUPPORT 59

INFANT BASIC LIFE SUPPORT 62
    FUNDAMENTALS 63
    AIRWAY MANAGEMENT 72
    AUTOMATED EXTERNAL DEFIBRILLATOR 80
    PERFORMING SINGLE-RESCUER INFANTBASIC LIFE SUPPORT 84
    PERFORMING 2-RESCUER INFANT BASICLIFE SUPPORT 88

AIRWAY MANAGEMENT 91
    REVIEW 92
    RESCUE BREATHING 96
    ADVANCED AIRWAY 98

CHOKING 100
    RELIEF OF ADULT CHOKING 102
    RELIEF OF CHILD CHOKING 105
    RELIEF OF INFANT CHOKING 108

ALTERNATE TOPICS 111
    MANAGEMENT OF OPIOID-INDUCEDEMERGENCY 112
    TEAM SYNCHRONY 116

UNIT 1:
ADULT BASIC LIFE SUPPORT

CHAPTER 1:
FUNDAMENTALS

BLS has a singular focus: restore normal heart and respiratory function. When BLS is indicated for someone experiencing cardiac arrest, the heart is no longer beating properly. It has either stopped beating completely (asystole) or is in a state of electrical malfunction that fails to produce cardiac output (ventricular fibrillation [VF], pulseless ventricular tachycardia [VT], or pulseless electrical activity [PEA]). Regardless of which abnormal heart rhythm the person is experiencing, BLS is the "cornerstone of resuscitation" and restoration of normal heart function (Meaney et al., 2013, p. 418). The same can be said for restoration of normal respiratory function. Let's identify the fundamentals of adult BLS, including environmental safety, initial assessment, emergency response system contact, 10-second check, and chest compressions.

Environmental Safety

The first step in adult BLS is confirming environmental safety. This safety check can provide crucial information about the scene and prevents undue harm to you or other rescuers (AHA, 2016). The American Red Cross recommends carefully inspecting the environment for potential hazards, including toxic debris, rapid water, smoke, traffic, live electrical wires, unsteady structures, or severe weather (2011). If the environment is deemed hazardous, then you should seek safety and alert emergency personnel of an identified victim and their location (ARC, 2011). If the environment is deemed safe, you should approach the victim while maintaining situational awareness.

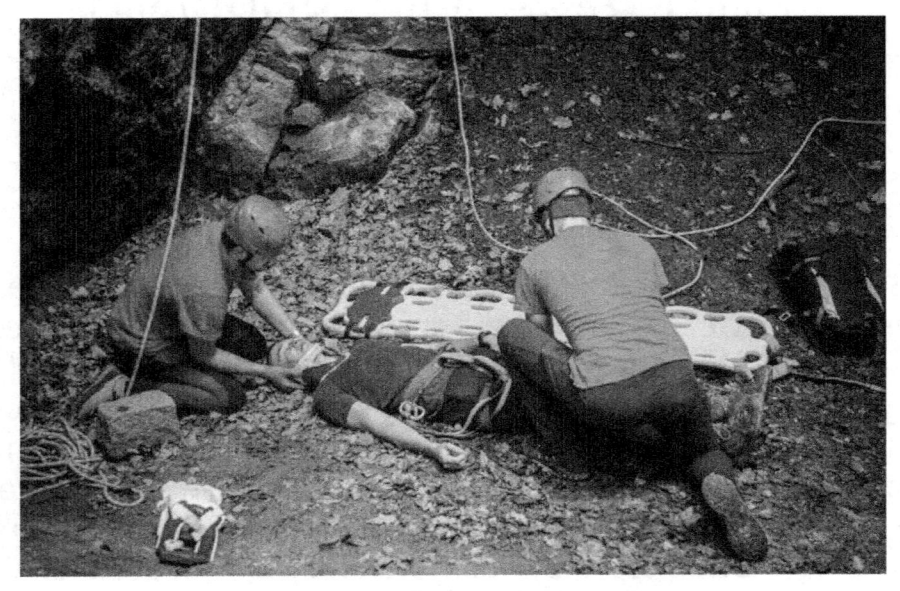

Image 1.

There are certain circumstances that necessitate moving the victim to a safe place before performing BLS. For example, a victim who is lying in a large puddle of water will need to be moved to a dry location because BLS often involves the use of an AED. Furthermore, using an AED while the victim is in water could cause harm to rescuers because of electrical conduction (University of Missouri, n.d.). A victim on snow or in a small amount of water does not need to be moved prior to AED use; however, water droplets present on the victim's chest need to be dried (AHA, 2016).

In addition to environmental safety, you must ensure personal safety by donning the correct personal protective equipment (PPE) before touching any bodily fluids. This prevents unnecessary exposure and potential transmission of blood-borne illnesses.

While donning the appropriate PPE, you can quickly inspect the victim's primary injury or problem. This allows you to prioritize and optimize rescue efforts. For example, you would be demonstrating poor prioritization if you became focused on stabilizing a dislocated ankle instead of addressing a victim's agonal breathing. You must prioritize and treat according to the primary threat to the victim's survival (Thim et al., 2012).

Initial Assessment

After the environment is considered safe or the victim is moved to a safe area, you must perform an initial assessment. This begins with assessing the victim's responsiveness. Consider using this approach:

- Kneel beside the victim.
- Place your hand on the victim's shoulder. Simultaneously shake the shoulder and shout to awaken the victim.
- A rapid assessment tool, AVPU (Alert, Verbal, Pain, Unresponsive), can provide additional information about the victim's level of consciousness (LOC). A response which is easily elicited indicates the victim is alert. A response that requires a verbal stimulus indicates a slightly decreased LOC. A response that requires a painful stimulus indicates a moderately decreased LOC. An unresponsive victim does not respond to any type of stimulus, cueing you to initiate BLS protocol.

After the victim's LOC is established, you can proceed based on immediate need. For the purposes of this guide, we will assume the victim is unresponsive and requires BLS.

Emergency Response System Contact

A lone rescuer needs assistance in an emergency. This is true for hospital and non-hospital settings. You should shout for help in either setting. When assistance arrives, you should direct that person to retrieve emergency equipment, such as an AED. If assistance is unavailable, you should leave the victim to retrieve emergency equipment (AHA, 2016).

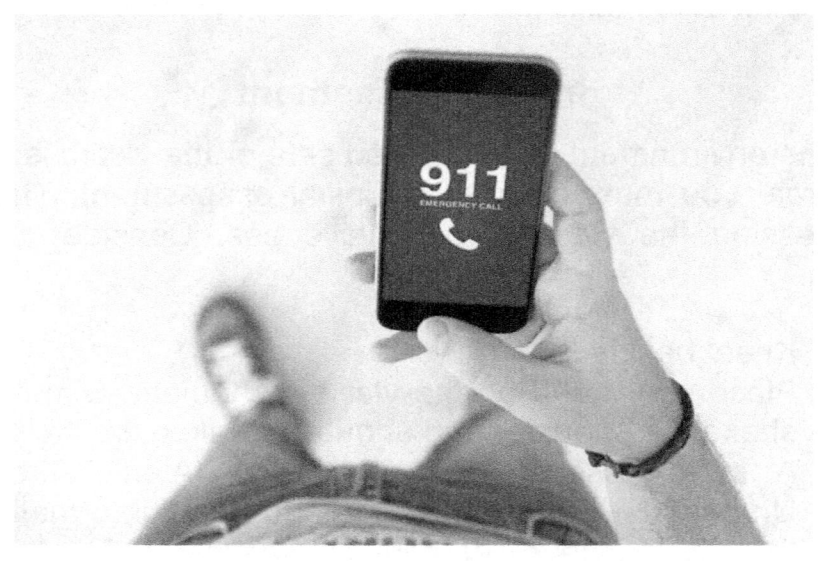

Image 2.

Technology can be very useful in BLS scenarios because of hands-free options. When initiating contact with the emergency response system (e.g.,, dialing 9-1-1), it is paramount to place the device on speakerphone to allow freedom of both hands for continued resuscitation efforts.

If in a hospital setting, shout for nearby help or activate the hospital's emergency response system (e.g., press the code blue button). Often, the hospital's phone system has a specific code that can be entered to override the phone system and notify the operator of an emergency. When speaking with the operator, it is crucial to give the victim's location and type of emergency assistance needed.

For example, you can tell the operator, "Code blue, hospital lobby, women's restroom." This will initiate the hospital's emergency response team, which often includes designated team members from anesthesia, critical care (provider and registered nurses), respiratory therapy, and laboratory. If the victim is experiencing an acute stroke, radiology will be called to attend the code. Predesignated, experienced code teams allow for smooth assessment and immediate intervention. Without code team designation, a rush of responders would cause chaos, incite confusion, and hamper resuscitation efforts.

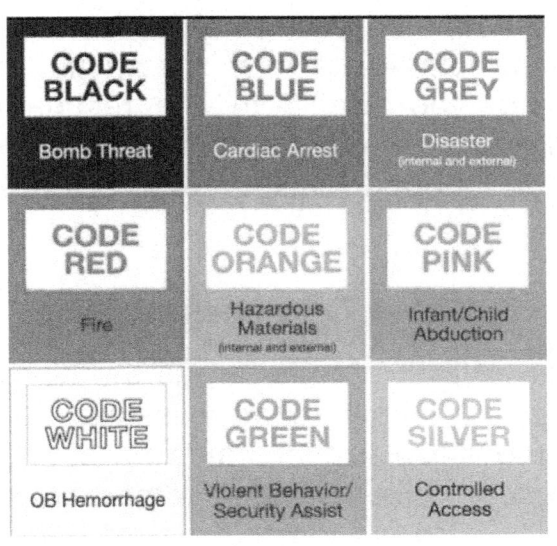

CODE BLACK	CODE BLUE	CODE GREY
Bomb Threat	Cardiac Arrest	Disaster (internal and external)
CODE RED	CODE ORANGE	CODE PINK
Fire	Hazardous Materials (internal and external)	Infant/Child Abduction
CODE WHITE	CODE GREEN	CODE SILVER
OB Hemorrhage	Violent Behavior/ Security Assist	Controlled Access

Image 3.

Healthcare workers must become familiar with their institution's emergency procedures and protocols. This optimizes patient safety and emergency responses. A color-coded chart may be offered at some institutions. These are often required to be placed within sight or on an employee's badge. Different colors designate the emergency and signal specific personnel to respond.

10-Second Check

The next critical step merges two assessments: pulse and breathing. Conducting these assessments simultaneously enables you to begin BLS without delay. In an adult victim, place two fingers on the victim's carotid artery while watching for inspiration or expiration. Avoid using the thumb, as this can cause you to mistakenly detect your own pulse. Never palpate both carotid arteries at the same time as this will obstruct blood flow to the brain. In total, this assessment should be completed within 10 seconds (AHA, 2016). This step is often referred to as "Look, listen, and feel" (Schlesinger, 2011).

If the victim is determined to be pulseless and not breathing, CPR should be initiated immediately. If the victim has a pulse but abnormal breathing, you should initiate rescue breathing. If the victim has a pulse and is breathing normally, remain beside the victim and provide support until emergency help arrives (AHA, 2016).

Chest Compressions

One component of BLS stands out as the single most important part of resuscitation—chest compressions. Simply put, chest compressions pump blood to the brain and other vital organs, and survival is *directly* linked with compression quality. Poor compression quality is "a preventable harm" and can decrease the rate of survival by as much as 30% (Meaney et al., 2013, p. 418).

For an adult victim, follow these steps:

- Kneel beside the victim. If the victim is in a bed or on a patient stretcher, get in the bed/stretcher or stand on a stool that allows you to provide chest compressions.
- *Optional:* Remove the victim's clothing to allow for proper inspection of anatomical locations (for example, the breastbone) and prepare for AED arrival.

- Place the heel of one hand in the middle of the victim's chest (the lower part of the breastbone) while interlocking the other hand on top (AHA, 2016).
- If unable to interlock hands, place one heel on the lower part of the breastbone while wrapping the other hand around the planted wrist.
- Keep both arms straight and place your body directly over your hands.
- Compress firmly by at least 2 inches on an adult victim.
- Complete at least 100-120 compressions per minute. To keep pace, compress to the tune of "Stayin' Alive" by the Bee Gees (AHA, 2020).
- Stay committed to continual compressions and avoid interruptions. This keeps blood flowing through the heart and to the rest of the body. Any interruption interferes with the victim's survival.
- Ensure the chest re-expands or recoils completely between each compression. Without full expansion, the heart and brain are not perfused properly and the victim's mean arterial pressure (MAP) declines (Yannopoulos et al., 2005).
- Ensure the victim is on a firm surface. A soft surface will absorb the compression effort and render the compressions ineffective. A firm surface opposes the compression force, thereby allowing a complete compression and perfusion (AHA, 2016).
- In an ideal situation, there should be at least 2 rescuers, and they should switch every two minutes. Providing chest compressions is very tiring, and rest periods are crucial for rescuers to provide quality compressions (AHA, 2016).

Here is a simplified version:

- Kneel beside the victim.

- Place the heel of one hand in the middle of the victim's chest with the other hand interlocked.
- Keep your arms straight and compress with your body directly over the victim.
- Compress at least 2 inches.
- Complete 100-120 compressions per minute.
- Allow full chest expansion between compressions.
- Do not stop until AED arrival.

Adult BLS Fundamentals Review

Let's review what we just learned and select three key points from each section to commit to memory.

Environmental safety

1. Before approaching the victim, scan the environment for safety concerns.
2. Protect yourself from injury or illness by donning the correct PPE.
3. If the victim is in an unsafe environment, move the victim to a safe location if it does not place either of you in danger.

Initial assessment

1. Assess the victim's responsiveness.
2. Shake the victim's shoulder and shout to awaken the victim.
3. Use the AVPU assessment tool to determine LOC.

Emergency response system contact

1. Regardless of setting, shout for help.
2. Use speakerphone to dial 9-1-1.

3. In a hospital, activate a code according to the institution's emergency protocols.

10-second check

1. Place two fingers (not the thumb) on the victim's carotid artery (not bilaterally).
2. Watch the victim's chest for expiration or inspiration during pulse check.
3. Complete these steps simultaneously within 10 seconds.

Chest compressions

1. Ensure the victim is on a firm surface.
2. Kneel beside the victim, straighten your arms, and lean over the victim's body.
3. Compress at least 2 inches at a rate of 100-120 compressions/minute while allowing chest re-expansion between each compression.

CHAPTER 2:
AIRWAY MANAGEMENT

The airway can be challenging to manage because every victim's anatomy is slightly different. The first goal in airway management during adult BLS is to open the airway. There are two maneuvers that facilitate airway opening and allow for oxygen delivery.

Maneuver 1 – Head Tilt–Chin Lift

The first maneuver is the most performed airway technique for an unresponsive victim. It is called the *head tilt–chin lift* and should only be performed on a victim who *does not* have a potential neck or head injury (AHA, 2016). After placing one hand on the victim's forehead, apply pressure to tilt the victim's head toward the ground. Next, take your other hand and position your fingers underneath the victim's chin. Lastly, pull the chin upward to open the airway and shift the tongue out of the way (AHA, 2016). A depiction of this maneuver is demonstrated in Image 4.

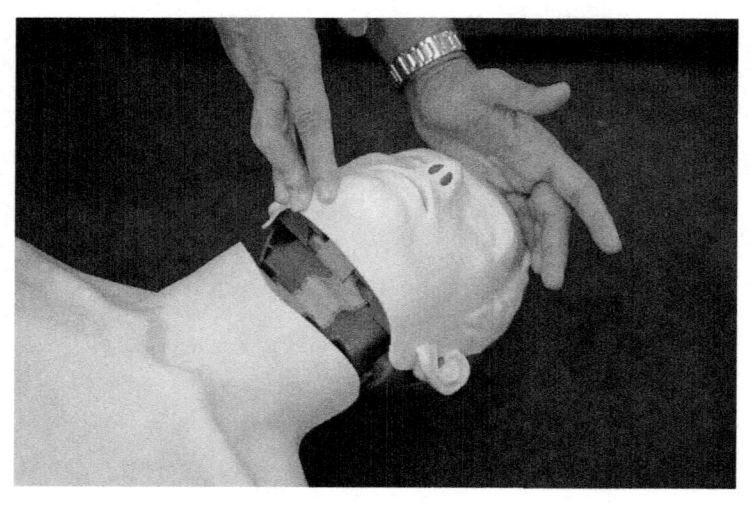

Image 4.

Avoid pressing into the soft tissue at the anterior of the neck (AHA, 2016). This can create further oxygenation issues and hamper obstruction relief attempts. An example of compression on the anterior neck's soft tissue can be seen in Image 5.

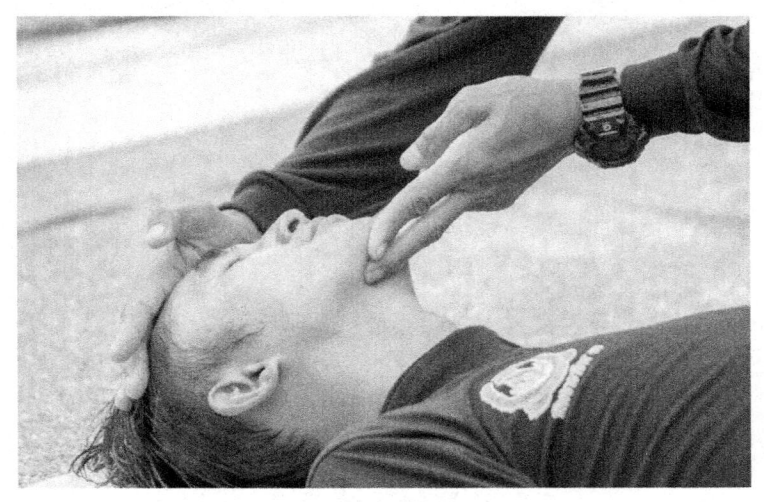

Image 5.

Maneuver 2 – Jaw Thrust

The second maneuver for those with airway issues—and potential head or neck injuries— is the jaw thrust. This maneuver takes adequate strength and two hands to complete; therefore, one rescuer will perform the jaw thrust while the other delivers oxygen (AHA, 2016). If this maneuver does not open the airway, you can switch to the head–tilt chin lift if the airway is obstructed.

First, stand directly behind the victim's head and place your elbows on the area behind the victim's head so that your hands can comfortably reach the jaw area (AHA, 2016). Next, "Place your fingers under the angles of the victim's lower jaw and lift with both hands, displacing the jaw forward" (AHA, 2016, p. 22). This allows you to relieve an obstruction and open the airway. See Image 6 for correct technique. It is important to ensure the mouth does not close, and if it does, position the mouth open by pressing the chin downward (AHA, 2016).

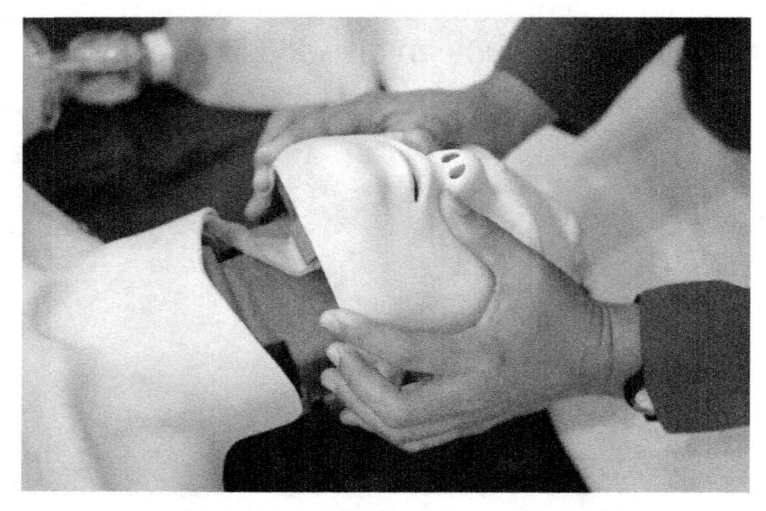

Image 6.

Adult Rescue Breathing

If, as a rescuer, you determine the pediatric victim has a pulse present but abnormal breathing, rescue breathing is appropriate. It is important to differentiate abnormal breathing from agonal gasps because agonal gasps can signal impending cardiac arrest; furthermore, presence of agonal gasps should prompt you to begin cardiopulmonary resuscitation (AHA, 2016). Two oxygen delivery devices are primarily used in BLS: a pocket mask and bag-valve mask.

Device 1 – Pocket Mask

Pocket masks have replaced face shields because they're associated with decreased rates of infection transmission (AHA, 2016). This type of mask is available for civilians to purchase in case of emergency. They can also be found in all medical settings that are equipped with first aid gear (see Image 7).

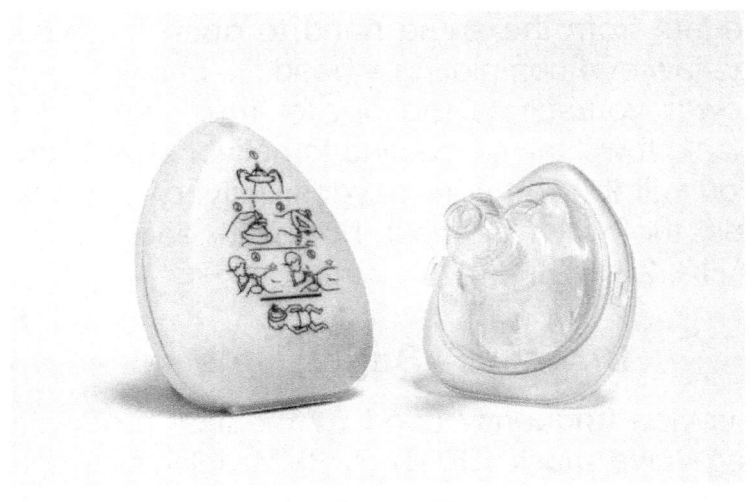

Image 7.

A pocket mask comes in different sizes: adult, child, and infant. Most pocket masks are equipped with a one-way valve that ensures fluid expelled from the victim is not directed toward the rescuer (AHA, 2016). This valve changes the direction of the victim's expiratory air and all secretions or vomit (AHA, 2016). The top of the mask has an opening that allows you to breathe into the mask for oxygen delivery. It is important to familiarize yourself with this device and become comfortable placing it on a victim's face.

To correctly place a pocket mask, kneel or stand to the side of the victim. The "pointy" end of the pocket mask fits over the victim's nose with the wide part below the mouth. The mask should be pressed firmly against the victim's face so that a seal is created. This seal can be made using the following method:

1. Use the index finger and thumb on the hand that is closest to the top of the victim to form a "C" shape around the air inlet. Your fingers should create a seal that prevents air leakage around the nose.
2. Use the thumb of your opposite hand to compress the lower portion of the face mask to the victim's face. Use the

fingers from the same hand to open the airway by lifting the jaw and completing a head tilt–chin lift.
3. Lower yourself to the pocket mask and breath into the mask. It will take 1 second to deliver an effective breath.
4. You will know if your oxygen delivery was effective if you see the victim's chest rise with each delivered breath (AHA, 2016).

Device 2 – Bag Valve Mask

Another device frequently used by medical professionals during BLS is a bag-valve mask (BVM). A BVM delivers ample oxygen to victims who are apneic or breathing abnormally. This device can be used while attached to oxygen or without supplemental oxygen. If used with oxygen, the BVM will deliver 100% oxygen; without an oxygen supply, the BVM delivers 21% oxygen, which is the amount of oxygen present in the air (AHA, 2016).

The name denotes exactly what the device comprises: a bag, a valve, and a mask. The bag is usually self-inflating, and the valve is non-rebreathing. This means the victim receives the appropriate amount of oxygenation and does not inhale carbon dioxide. This mask differs from the pocket mask because it has more cushion and the ability to provide a snug fit around the nose and mouth. This design prevents air leakage. Both masks and bags vary in size to fit adults, children, and infants.

It is important to locate the oxygen inlet on the opposite end of the mask to connect oxygen supply when needed. In Image 8, oxygen tubing is already connected to the inlet. Another key part of the BVM is the reservoir bag. This bag allows for high concentrations of oxygen to be maintained with BVM use; each time the bag is compressed, it fills with highly concentrated oxygen instead of room air containing 21% oxygen (AHA, 2016). The reservoir bag can also be seen in its deflated form in Image 8.

Proper use of the BVM begins with positioning. Begin by standing or kneeling above the victim's head. Next, use the E-C method to ensure a tight seal around the victim's nose and mouth. This technique is best performed with two rescuers, but it can be performed with one as well. Steps for single-rescuer BVM use include:

1. Place the mask on the victim's face with the "pointy" end over the nose and the wider portion below the mouth. Pull the bag toward the side you will be compressing while ensuring the bag is perpendicular to the victim's body. Keep the bag level so that the air supply is not cut off.
2. Form a "C" shape with your thumb and index finger and wrap around the mask, keeping close to the edge.
3. Form an "E" with your middle, ring, and pinky fingers, and lift the jaw upward. This mimics a head tilt–chin lift.
4. While ensuring a tight seal with one hand, use the other hand to compress the bag. It is unnecessary to forcefully squeeze the bag as this can cause increased intrathoracic pressure over time.
5. A slow, steady squeeze will deliver an effective breath. You will know if your oxygen delivery was effective if you see the victim's chest rise with each compression of the bag (AHA, 2016).

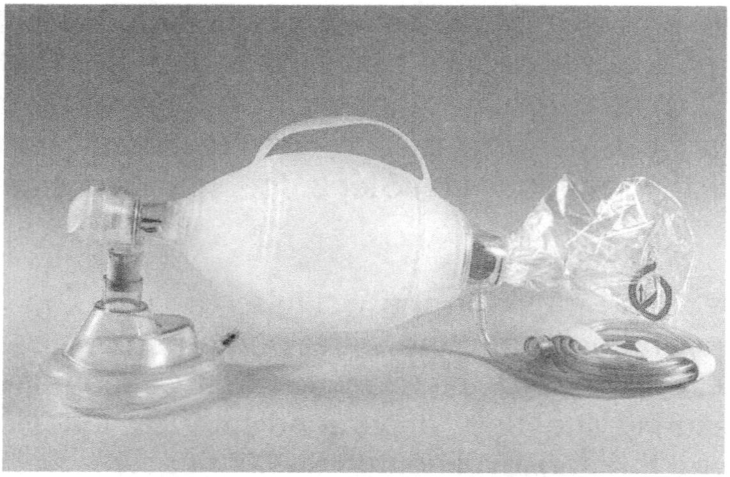

Image 8.

2-rescuer BVM use is the preferred method because the victim will receive higher quality ventilation. While your partner uses both hands to ensure the mask is completely sealed to the victim's face, can compress the bag to deliver the breath, or vice versa. More detailed steps include:

1. Your partner will stand above the victim's head and position the mask over the victim's face while you stand to the side of the victim.
2. Using the aforementioned "EC" method, your partner seals the mask to the victim's face on one side and then mirrors this technique on the other side. This ensures a complete, circumferential seal.
3. You can now squeeze the bag to deliver a breath at a slow, steady rate.

Unavailable Equipment

If equipment is unavailable for the provision of airway support (e.g., pocket mask or BVM), there are other practices that can be implemented to provide breaths. Although these practices increase the risk for disease or infection transmission, they can be life-saving interventions for some. The AHA encourages hands-only cardiopulmonary resuscitation (CPR) if airway equipment is unavailable (2020). However, whether or not to deliver rescue breaths is ultimately at your discretion. Here is how to properly perform mouth-to-mouth, an alternative strategy appropriate for adult victims:

1. Perform a head tilt–chin lift.
2. Use your index finger and thumb to close the victim's nose (AHA, 2016).
3. Make a seal with your mouth and provide one breath until you see the victim's chest rise (AHA, 2016).

CHAPTER 3:
AUTOMATED EXTERNAL DEFIBRILLATOR

An automated external defibrillator is a small, portable machine that may be found in various locations like hospitals, schools, factories, stores, or even homes (Mayo Clinic, 2020). This machine provides unsynchronized electrical shock to rhythms identified as shockable, such as ventricular fibrillation (VF) or pulseless ventricular tachycardia (pVT) (AHA, 2016; Zoll, n.d.). If the rhythm is not shockable, the AED will advise you to continue chest compressions without defibrillation (Mayo Clinic, 2020). Examples of non-shockable rhythms include pulseless electrical activity (PEA) and asystole.

Early defibrillation is the *best* chance at stopping the leading fatal rhythm encountered during BLS—ventricular fibrillation. Compressions alone are usually not effective in stopping VF (Gu & Chun-Sheng, 2016). The Mayo Clinic stresses the importance of early defibrillation and alludes to the brain and organ damage that can result from delayed defibrillation (2020). Therefore, as soon as the AED arrives at the scene, you should attach the electrodes to the victim and begin analyzing the victim's heart rhythm. The precise steps involved in AED use include include:

1. Place the AED beside the victim on the opposite side of the compressor. This allows you and another rescuer, if applicable, to complete your resuscitative efforts without interruption (AHA, 2016).
2. Open the AED and turn the machine on. Often, the AED will begin directing you through audible prompts. Listen closely to the steps.
3. Peel the backing off the provided electrodes/pads and adhere them to the victim's skin in the correct locations. There should be a visual diagram in the AED pack to

ensure correct placement. For an adult victim or anyone over the age of 8, place adult electrodes. This ensures enough voltage reaches the victim's heart. There are different locations for AED pad placement. Don't forget the main principle of pad placement: The heart must be in-between the pads because electric shock moves between them. Therefore, the first pad could be placed inferior to the right shoulder with the second pad on the left mid-axillary line (as shown in Image 9). Another option includes placing the first pad anterolateral and the second pad anteroposterior (AHA, 2016). If child electrodes are available only for an adult victim, it is best to continue chest compressions instead of shocking the adult victim with child electrodes. This is because the amount of electricity is not sufficient to reset an adult victim's arrhythmia (AHA, 2016).

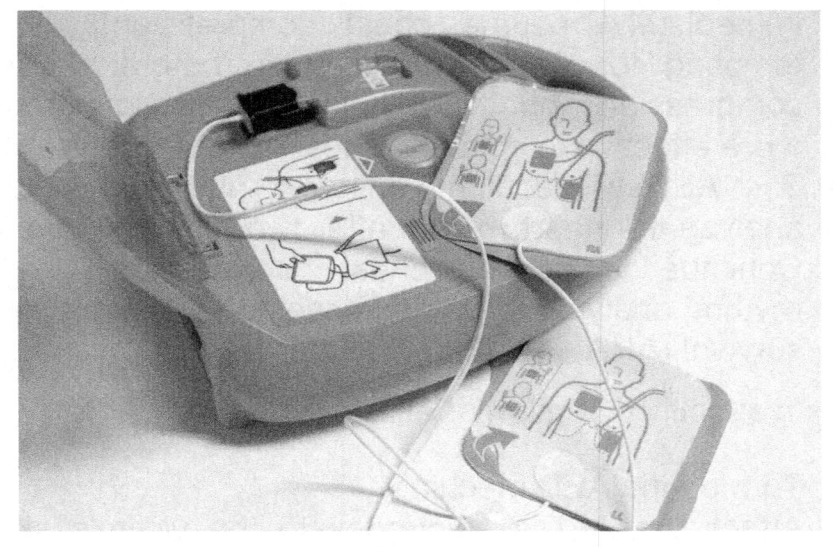

Image 9.

4. Plug the electrodes into the AED and wait for the next prompt from the machine. It will direct you to stop

compressions for a momentary analysis of the victim's heart rhythm. It is extremely important to stop compressions at this time to ensure proper heart rhythm analysis.
5. If the victim's heart rhythm is deemed shockable, the AED will prompt you to take all hands off the victim. A common term for this step is to "clear" the victim (AHA, 2016).

    a. Recent evidence suggests that there are benefits to completing compressions in between heart rhythm analysis and shock. This optimizes coronary perfusion and increases the chance for survival (AHA, 2016).

6. Ensure everyone is clear of the victim (including the person delivering breaths) before pressing the shock button.
7. Once you press the shock button, the compressor should immediately resume chest compressions. It may be tempting to palpate for a pulse before starting chest compressions, but this will hinder resuscitation efforts. It is more effective to continue chest compressions.
8. The AED will continue to work and advise you to re-analyze the heart rhythm after two minutes have elapsed. Continue to provide chest compressions in between rhythm analysis. This increases the victim's chance of survival (AHA, 2016).

Here is a simplified version of AED use:

1. Turn on the AED machine.
2. Attach the AED's electrodes to the victim's skin in the correct locations.
3. Plug the electrodes into the AED machine.

4. Press the analyze button to determine if the rhythm is shockable.
5. Direct all rescuers to remove their hands from the victim.
6. Press the shock button if the rhythm is shockable.
7. Immediately restart chest compressions.

Exceptional Conditions

Under certain conditions, there may be additional considerations that you should take prior to using an AED. Therefore, it's important to pay attention to each unique victim and assess the situation for possible obstacles.

When removing a victim's clothing to expose the chest for placement of AED electrodes, you should note whether the victim has a large amount of chest hair. Chest hair can impede heart rhythm analysis and prevent the AED from effectively delivering shock. For this reason, you'll need to either shave the areas before electrode placement or utilize one set of pads to "wax" them. The waxing technique should only be done if there is a second set of electrodes in the AED kit (AHA, 2016).

Like chest hair, medication patches that are adhered to the victim's skin can impede an AED's electrical shock. In addition, AED electrodes placed on top of them can produce minor burns. Medication patches must be removed prior to placement of AED pads to avoid these consequences. Before removing the patch, however, don gloves to ensure the medication is not transferred to your skin with removal. For example, if you were to touch a nitroglycerin patch without gloves, it could cause acute hypotension, headache, and dizziness (Mayo Clinic, 2021). Once you have gloves on, take the medication patch off and wipe the area to remove any remaining medication. The patch should be placed in a sharps container to prevent accidental exposure to others or the environment.

Implanted cardiac defibrillators and pacemakers are usually easy to detect because of their prominent figure. The most common location is the upper chest (see Image 10). If an AED electrode is placed over one of these devices, electrical shock will be prevented from reaching the heart. Therefore, you must place the electrodes to the side, above, or below the device to ensure proper energy delivery. It is critical to place the electrodes so that the victim's heart is in between the pads. This allows for electrical conduction to reach the heart.

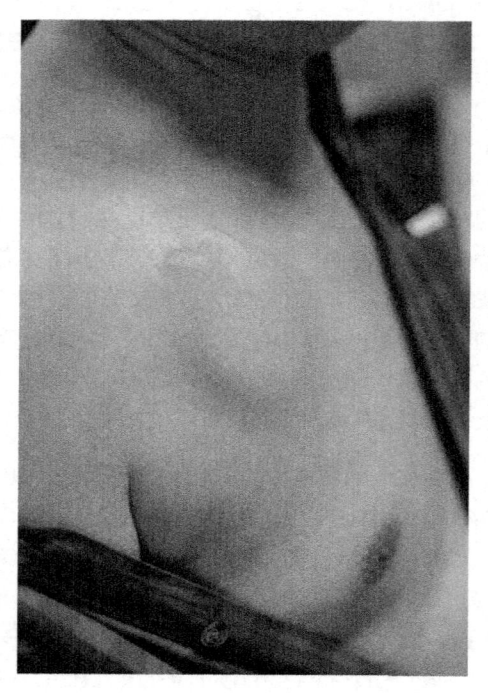

Image 10.

CHAPTER 4:
PERFORMING SINGLE-RESCUER ADULT BASIC LIFE SUPPORT

Let's combine the individual tools of BLS and review how to perform Single-Rescuer Adult BLS. Before we begin, think back to the main concepts of adult BLS:

1. Ensuring environmental safety
2. Performing an initial assessment
3. Contacting the emergency response system
4. Completing a 10-second check
5. Performing chest compressions
6. Managing the victim's airway
7. Using the AED

Scenario

It's Sunday evening. You stop at the local grocery store to pick up a few items for the upcoming week. The store is closing soon, so you quickly check out and head to your car. While walking through the parking lot, you see an older man next to his car, clutching his chest and groaning. He falls to the ground and stops making noise. What are your next steps?

Action

It is time to apply your knowledge of BLS and act! First, **inspect the environment to ensure the safety of yourself and the victim.** For example, if the victim were lying in the path of traffic, it would be necessary to move the victim to a safe location, such as the sidewalk. However, it is imperative to not place yourself in danger, so be mindful of traffic and your movements. Since it is evening, moving the victim to a safe location is especially important because of low visibility for drivers.

After confirming environmental safety, it is time to **perform an initial assessment** of the victim. Place your hand on the victim's shoulder. Simultaneously shake the shoulder and shout to see if the victim responds. Examples of what to shout include "Are you there?" or "Can you open your eyes?" The AVPU tool can further help classify the victim's LOC. While completing this initial assessment, you quickly scan the victim's body for any other obvious injury, but you see nothing abnormal.

The victim remains unresponsive to your attempts at awakening or eliciting a response. Therefore, you begin to **yell for help**. You see no one else in the parking lot, so you run to the grocery store to obtain emergency equipment like an AED. While on your way, you pull out your cell phone and dial 9-1-1 while on speakerphone. This action **initiates contact with the emergency response system**. The manager meets you at the entrance of the store, and you direct him to get an AED for an unresponsive patron in the parking lot.

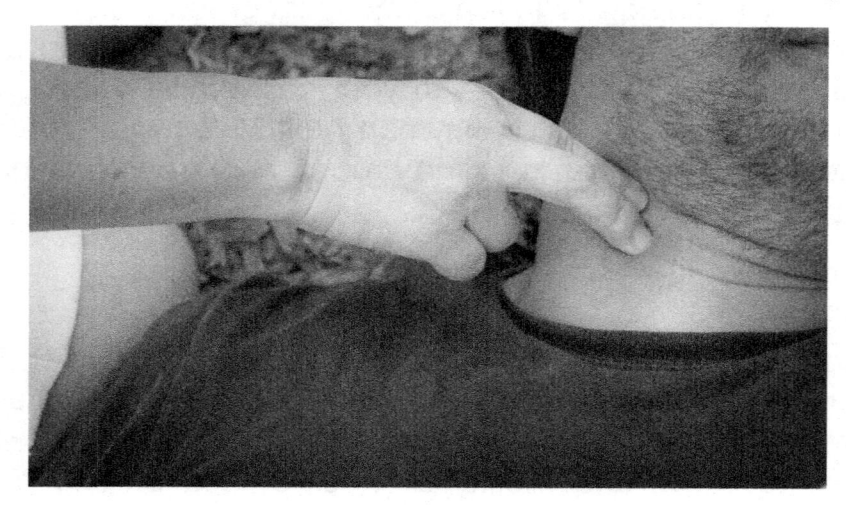

Image 11.

You quickly return to the victim and begin performing a **10-second check**. You place two fingers on the carotid artery as seen in Image 11. You are careful to not use your thumb because of the potential to feel your own pulse. As you are palpating for the presence of a pulse, you closely watch the victim's chest for any sign of inspiration or expiration. You determine, within 10 seconds, that he does not have a palpable pulse and has agonal breathing. He is gasping for air and making occasional snoring sounds. You recognize this type of breathing as abnormal and as an ominous sign of cardiac arrest (AHA, 2016).

In addition to agonal breathing, you understand the absence of a pulse indicates blood has stopped flowing to the heart, brain, and other vital organs. It is now time to begin **chest compressions**. As you quickly remove the victim's shirt (e.g., tearing if necessary), you locate his breastbone, place one heel of the hand on the lower part of the breastbone and interlock the other hand on top. While keeping your arms straight and leaning over his body, you compress at a rate of 100-120 compressions per minute. You hum the tune of "Stayin' Alive" to keep pace.

You notice the chest is not fully re-expanding with each compression, so you correct this technique while ensuring you compress 2 inches. You remember that full chest re-expansion is imperative for maintaining cardiac perfusion. After 30 compressions pass, you decide to continue with chest compressions only. Without an available pocket mask, you feel uncomfortable **providing airway support**. This is appropriate because, according to the AHA, "Hands-Only CPR has been shown to be as effective as conventional CPR for cardiac arrest at home, at work or in public" (2020, para. 3). You recall that with a pocket mask, the compression-to-ventilation ratio for single-rescuer BLS is 30 compressions to 2 breaths (AHA, 2016).

As a few minutes pass, you start to become tired, but you remind yourself how important chest compressions are for the victim's survival. Finally, help arrives. For this scenario, let's suppose the help is not knowledgeable of BLS. Therefore, you must play multiple roles until emergency personnel arrive.

Now that **you have an AED**, you quickly open the device and turn on the machine. The device prompts you to place the pads on the victim's skin. You notice a large bump in the right chest wall and assume it is an implanted defibrillator or pacemaker. Careful to avoid placing a pad on this area, you place the pad below the device. You place the second pad in the left mid-axillary line to ensure the heart is between the pads. As the AED analyzes the victim's rhythm, you remain clear of the victim. Shock is advised, so you resume chest compressions until it is time to press the shock button. Before pressing the button, you make sure no one is touching the victim. Immediately after pressing the shock button, you restart quality chest compressions. You still don't have a pocket mask for managing the airway, so you continue chest compressions until the AED re-analyzes the heart rhythm.

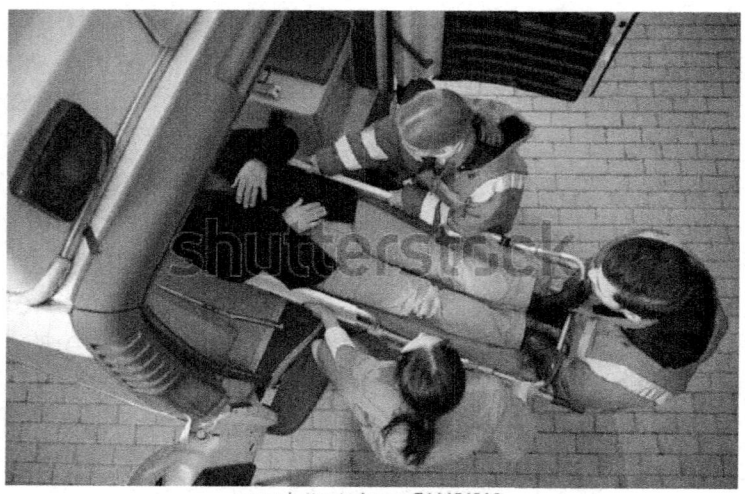

Image 12.

An ambulance arrives and the emergency personnel take over chest compressions. After one more unsynchronized defibrillation, the victim restores an organized heart rhythm! Emergency personnel transport the victim to a nearby hospital that has cardiac catheter capability.

CHAPTER 5:
PERFORMING 2-RESCUER ADULT BASIC LIFE SUPPORT

Now, let's assess a different scenario and discuss the appropriate actions when 2 rescuers are available to provide BLS. Before we begin, let's review the main concepts of adult BLS one more time:

1. Ensuring environmental safety
2. Performing an initial assessment
3. Contacting the emergency response system
4. Completing a 10-second check
5. Performing chest compressions
6. Managing the victim's airway
7. Using the AED

Scenario

You are an emergency medical technician (EMT) on duty with a partner. It's lunchtime, so you and your partner stop at a fast food restaurant for a quick bite to eat. When entering the restaurant, you hear commotion and see a small crowd standing around a young adult male lying on the floor. The crowd motions for you to approach the victim. You both spring into action and begin BLS efforts. What should you do first?

Action

Before approaching the victim, it is crucial to **verify environmental safety**. Consider reasons for the victim's collapse that may make the environment unsafe. Examples include violence, toxic chemicals, or a gas leak. You rule out these factors and both approach the victim to begin resuscitative efforts.

Your partner **begins the initial assessment** by shaking the teenager's shoulder and shouting, "Are you there?" No response from the victim indicates unresponsiveness and warrants **contacting the emergency response system**. Luckily, you *are* the emergency response system, so backup is dependent upon your preference/situation. You have all the necessary equipment for resuscitation and see no additional victims. You decide not to call for further backup. Depending on protocol, it is the EMT's responsibility to contact the receiving hospital of the victim at the proper time, such as when the ambulance is actively en route.

You place two fingers between the victim's trachea and neck muscles to determine the presence of a carotid pulse (AHA, 2016). This is **completed in 10 seconds** while scanning the victim's chest for inspiration or expiration. Assessment reveals pulselessness and apnea.

After communicating the assessment to your partner, you use scissors to tear the victim's shirt open to expose the chest and **begin chest compressions**. You compress at a rate of 100-120 compressions per minute and at a depth of 2 inches. The heel of one hand is on the lower part of the victim's breastbone with the other hand interlocked. Ensuring your arms are straight and body leaned over the victim's body, the victim's chest re-expands between each compression for optimal cardiac perfusion. You recognize the surface underneath the victim (concrete floor) is appropriate resistance for chest compressions.

Your partner runs to the ambulance to retrieve airway equipment and an AED. When he returns, you have completed 30 compressions, so your partner provides two breaths with a bag-valve mask. After the breaths have been provided, you continue chest compressions while your partner attaches the AED pads to the victim. The AED begins to analyze the victim's heart rhythm. Both of you remain clear of the victim. Shock is indicated; therefore, you begin chest compressions while the AED charges. Your partner states, "Everyone clear!" You take your hands off the victim and ensure no equipment is touching him. After your partner presses the shock button, you immediately resume chest compressions at a rate of 30 compressions to 2 breaths.

After two minutes, the AED re-analyzes the victim's heart rhythm and determines the rhythm is not shockable. Your partner checks for a carotid pulse and palpates a weak, but present, pulse. The victim starts to move slightly. The victim's arrythmia has been successfully converted to an organized rhythm; therefore, you can immediately begin post-cardiac arrest care (return of spontaneous circulation [ROSC]) by applying oxygen, taking a set of vital signs, and preparing for transfer to a hospital setting.

UNIT 2:
PEDIATRIC BASIC LIFE SUPPORT

There are important differences between adult BLS and pediatric BLS. Before BLS efforts begin on a potential pediatric victim, you must quickly confirm age through assessment. A victim is considered a child if they're between the age of 1 and the start of puberty (AHA, 2016). To determine if the child has reached puberty, assess for "breast development in females and the presence of axillary hair in males" (Topjian et al., 2020, p. 3).

Early, effective BLS significantly improves the survival rate for children who suffer respiratory distress or cardiac arrest (AHA, 2016). This is evidenced by the 19% increase in survival rate for children who experienced cardiac arrest from 2000 to 2018 (Topjian et al., 2020). The importance of this topic cannot be overstated. Let's delve into this topic and discuss the specifics of pediatric BLS, including fundamentals, airway management, AED use, and rescuer actions.

CHAPTER 6:
FUNDAMENTALS

Pediatric BLS shares the same goal as adult BLS: restore normal heart and respiratory function. Topjian et al. report the incidence of cardiac arrest in children and infants reaches 20,000 annually (2020). This overwhelming number highlights the importance of BLS knowledge for medical professionals and bystanders. Let's discover the fundamentals of BLS for children, including environmental safety, initial assessment, emergency response system contact, 10-second check, and chest compressions.

Environmental Safety

The first step in pediatric BLS is confirming environmental safety. This safety check can provide crucial information about the scene and prevents undue harm to you or other rescuers (AHA, 2016). The American Red Cross recommends carefully inspecting the environment for potential hazards, including toxic debris, rapid water, smoke, traffic, live electrical wires, unsteady structures, or severe weather (2011). If the environment is deemed hazardous, then you should seek safety and alert emergency personnel of an identified victim and their location (ARC, 2011). If the environment is deemed safe, you should approach the victim while maintaining situational awareness.

There are certain circumstances that necessitate moving the victim to a safe place before performing BLS. For example, a victim who is lying in a large puddle of water will need to be moved to a dry location because BLS often involves the use of an AED. Furthermore, using an AED while the victim is in water could cause harm to rescuers because of electrical conduction (University of Missouri, n.d.). A victim on snow or in a small amount of water does not need to be moved prior to AED use; however, water droplets present on the child's chest need to be dried (AHA, 2016).

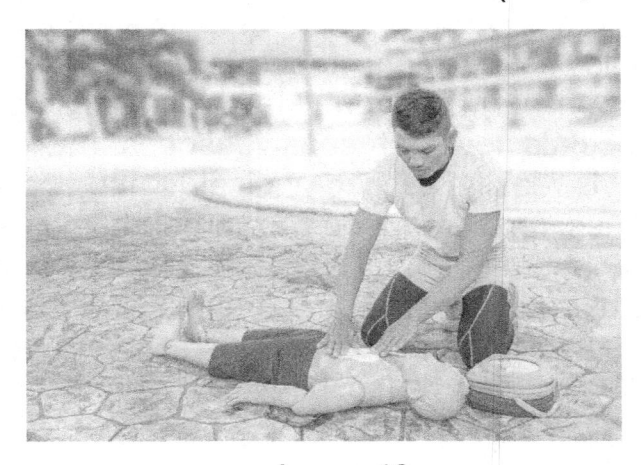

Image 13.

In addition to environmental safety, you must ensure personal safety by donning the correct personal protective equipment before touching any bodily fluids. This prevents unnecessary exposure and potential transmission of blood-borne illnesses.

While donning the appropriate PPE, you can quickly inspect the victim's primary injury or problem. This allows you to prioritize and optimize rescue efforts. For example, you would be demonstrating poor prioritization if you became focused on checking for pupillary response instead of treating the child's agonal breathing. You must prioritize and treat according to the primary threat to the victim's survival (Thim et al., 2012).

Initial Assessment

After the environment is considered safe or the victim is moved to a safe area, you must perform an initial assessment. This begins with assessing the victim's responsiveness. Consider using this approach:

- Kneel beside the victim.
- Place your hand on the victim's shoulder. Simultaneously shake the shoulder and shout to awaken the victim.
- A rapid assessment tool, AVPU (Alert, Verbal, Pain, Unresponsive), can provide additional information about the victim's level of consciousness (LOC). A response which is easily elicited indicates the victim is alert. A response that requires a verbal stimulus indicates a slightly decreased LOC. A response that requires a painful stimulus indicates a moderately decreased LOC. An unresponsive victim does not respond to any type of stimulus, cueing you to initiate BLS protocol.

After the victim's LOC is established, you can proceed based on immediate need. For the purposes of this guide, we will assume the victim is unresponsive and requires BLS.

Emergency Response System Contact

A lone rescuer needs assistance in an emergency. This is true for hospital and non-hospital settings. You should shout for help in either setting. When assistance arrives, you should direct that person to retrieve emergency equipment, such as an AED.

One key difference between adult and child BLS is the correct time to retrieve the AED if no assistance is available. To review, in adult BLS, you should immediately retrieve the AED if the victim is deemed unresponsive and you are unable to activate the emergency response system (e.g., no cell phone). In pediatric BLS, however, you must base your actions on whether the collapse was witnessed. If the collapse was witnessed and the child is unresponsive or pulseless (complete the 10-second check), leave the scene to immediately get the AED and initiate emergency response system contact (AHA, 2016). If the collapse was not witnessed and the child is unresponsive or pulseless (complete the

10-second check), you should perform sets of 30 chest compressions and 2 breaths for two minutes before leaving the scene to retrieve the AED and initiate contact with the emergency response system (AHA, 2016). To summarize, *in pediatric BLS, you may need to merge the step to contact the emergency response system contact and the 10-second check step depending on whether the collapse was witnessed.* Let's reiterate these key points:

- Witnessed collapse → If alone, leave to get the AED and initiate contact.
- Unwitnessed collapse → If alone, complete two minutes of chest compressions before leaving to get the AED and initiate contact.

Technology can be very useful in BLS scenarios because of hands-free options. When initiating contact with the emergency response system (e.g., dialing 9-1-1), it is paramount to place the device on speakerphone to allow freedom of both hands for continued resuscitation efforts.

If in a hospital setting, shout for nearby help or activate the hospital's emergency response system (e.g., press the code blue button). Often, the hospital's phone system has a specific code that can be entered to override the phone system and notify the operator of an emergency. When speaking with the operator, it is crucial to give the victim's location and type of emergency assistance needed.

For example, you can tell the operator, "Code blue, 3rd floor, room 325." This will initiate the hospital's emergency response team, which often includes designated team members from anesthesia, critical care (provider and registered nurses), respiratory therapy, and laboratory. If the victim is experiencing an acute stroke, radiology will be called to attend the code. Predesignated, experienced code teams allow for smooth assessment and immediate intervention. Without code team designation, a rush of responders would cause chaos, incite confusion, and hamper resuscitation efforts.

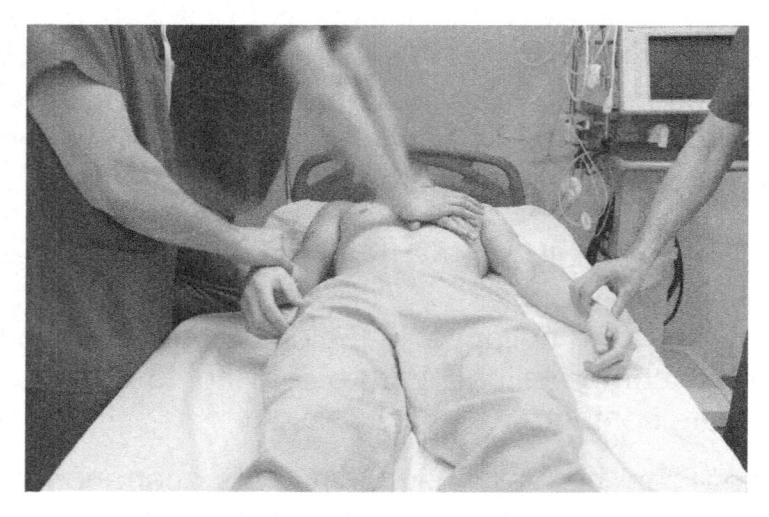

Image 14.

Healthcare workers must become familiar with their institution's emergency procedures and protocols. This optimizes patient safety and emergency responses. A color-coded chart may be offered at some institutions (see Image 3). These are often required to be placed within sight or on an employee's badge. Different colors designate the emergency and signal specific personnel to respond.

10-Second Check

The next critical step merges two assessments: pulse and breathing. Conducting these assessments simultaneously enables you to begin BLS without delay. *In pediatric BLS, you may need to merge the step to contact the emergency response system contact and the 10-second check step depending on whether the collapse was witnessed.* Place two fingers on the victim's carotid artery while watching for inspiration or expiration. Avoid using the thumb, as this can cause you to mistakenly detect your own pulse. Never palpate both carotid arteries at the same time as this will obstruct blood flow to the brain. If you can't locate the carotid pulse, the femoral pulse can also be palpated in children. This pulse is palpated "in the inner thigh, midway between the hip bone and the pubic bone" (AHA, 2016, p. 48). See Image 15 for reference. In total, assessing the child's breathing and pulse should be completed within 10 seconds (AHA, 2016). This step is often referred to as "Look, listen, and feel" (Schlesinger, 2011).

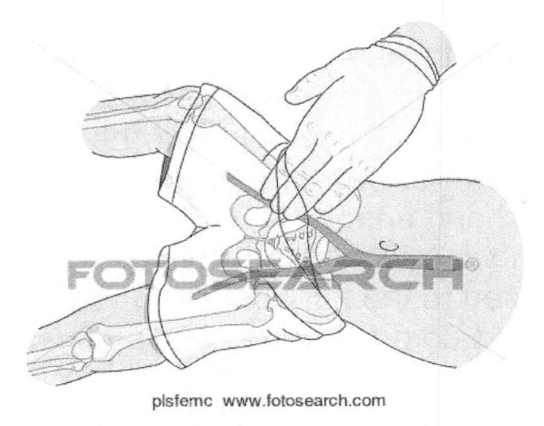

Image 15.

If the victim is determined to be pulseless and not breathing, CPR should be initiated immediately. If the victim has a pulse but abnormal breathing, you should initiate rescue breathing. If the victim has a pulse and is breathing normally, remain beside the victim and provide support until emergency help arrives (AHA, 2016).

Chest Compressions

One component of BLS stands out as the single most important part of resuscitation—chest compressions. Simply put, chest compressions pump blood to the brain and other vital organs, and survival is *directly* linked with compression quality. Poor compression quality is called "a preventable harm" and can decrease the rate of survival by as much as 30% (Meaney et al., 2013, p. 418).

For a pediatric victim, follow these steps:

- Kneel beside the victim. If the victim is in a bed or a patient stretcher, get in the bed/stretcher or stand on a stool that allows you to provide chest compressions.
- *Optional:* Remove the victim's clothing to allow for proper inspection of anatomical locations (for example, the breastbone) and prepare for AED arrival.
- Place the heel of one hand in the middle of the victim's chest (the lower part of the breastbone) while interlocking the other hand on top (AHA, 2016).
- One hand may be used instead of two if the chest is compressed to the right depth.
- You should compress the child's chest "at least one third the anteroposterior (AP) diameter of the chest (about 2 inches, or 5 cm) with each compression" (AHA, 2016, p. 50).
- Keep both arms straight and place your body directly over your hands.
- Complete at least 100-120 compressions per minute. To keep pace, compress to the tune of "Stayin' Alive" by the Bee Gees (AHA, 2020).
- Stay committed to continual compressions and avoid interruptions. This keeps blood flowing through the heart and to the rest of the body. Any interruption interferes with the victim's survival.
- Ensure the chest re-expands or recoils completely between each compression. Without full expansion, the heart and brain are not perfused properly and the victim's mean arterial pressure (MAP) declines (Yannopoulos et al., 2005).

- Ensure the victim is on a firm surface. A soft surface will absorb the compression effort and render the compressions ineffective. A firm surface opposes the compression force, thereby allowing a complete compression and perfusion (AHA, 2016).
- In an ideal situation, there should be at least 2 rescuers, and you should switch every two minutes. Providing chest compressions is very tiring, and rest periods are crucial for rescuers to provide quality compressions (AHA, 2016).

Here is a simplified version:

- Kneel beside the victim.
- Place the heel of one hand in the middle of the victim's chest with the other hand interlocked. You can use one hand only if you're able to compress to the proper depth.
- Keep your arms straight and compress with your body directly over the victim.
- Compress at least 2 inches or 1/3 the AP diameter of the child's chest (AHA, 2016).
- Complete 100-120 compressions per minute.
- Allow full chest expansion between compressions.
- Do not stop until AED arrival.

Pediatric BLS Fundamentals Review

Let's review what we just learned and select three key points from each section to commit to memory.

Environmental safety

1. Before approaching the child, scan the environment for safety concerns.
2. Protect yourself from injury or illness by donning the correct PPE.

3. If the victim is in an unsafe environment, move the child to a safe location if it does not place either of you in danger.

Initial assessment

1. Assess the child's responsiveness.
2. Shake the child's shoulder and shout to awaken.
3. Use the AVPU assessment tool to determine LOC.

Emergency response system contact

1. Regardless of setting, shout for help.
2. Use speakerphone to dial 9-1-1.
3. In pediatric BLS, you may need to modify and/or merge the step to contact the emergency response system and the 10-second check step depending on whether the collapse was witnessed.
    a. Witnessed collapse → If alone, leave to get the AED and initiate contact.
    b. Unwitnessed collapse → If alone, complete two minutes of chest compressions before leaving to get the AED and initiate contact.

10-second check

1. Place two fingers on the child's carotid or femoral artery.
2. Watch chest for expiration or inspiration during pulse check.
3. Complete these steps simultaneously within 10 seconds.

Chest compressions

1. Ensure the victim is on a firm surface.

2. Kneel beside the victim, straighten arms, and lean over the victim's body.
3. Compress at least 2 inches (or 1/3 the AP diameter of the chest) at a rate of 100-120 compressions/minute while allowing chest re-expansion between each compression (AHA, 2016).

CHAPTER 7:
AIRWAY MANAGEMENT

The airway can be challenging to manage because every victim's anatomy is slightly different. Like adult BLS, the first goal in airway management during pediatric BLS is to open the airway. There are two maneuvers that facilitate airway opening and allow for oxygen delivery.

Maneuver 1 – Head Tilt–Chin Lift

The first maneuver is the most performed airway technique for an unresponsive child. It is called the *head tilt–chin lift* and should only be performed on a child who *does not* have a potential neck or head injury (AHA, 2016). After placing one hand on the victim's forehead, apply pressure to tilt the victim's head toward the ground. Next, take your other hand and position your fingers underneath the victim's chin. Lastly, pull the chin upward to open the airway and shift the tongue out of the way (AHA, 2016). A depiction of this maneuver is demonstrated in Image 16. Avoid pressing into the soft tissue at the anterior of the neck (AHA, 2016). This can create further oxygenation issues and hamper obstruction relief attempts.

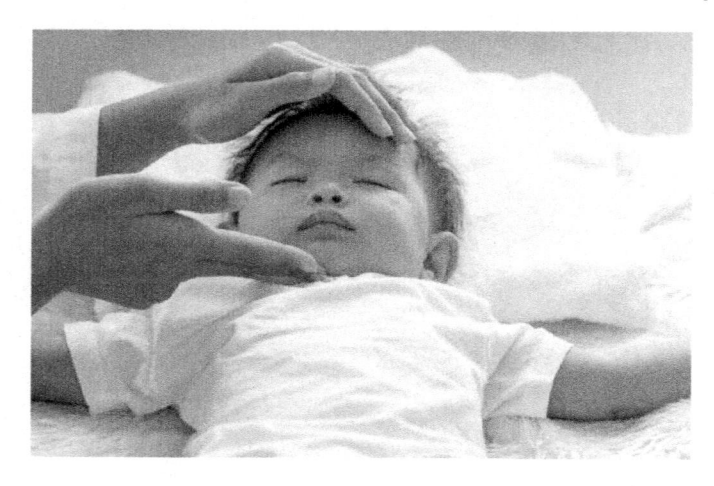

Image 16.

Maneuver 2 – Jaw Thrust

As with adult BLS, the second maneuver that can be implemented for children with airway issues (and victims with potential head or neck injuries) is the jaw thrust. This maneuver takes adequate strength and two hands to complete; therefore, one rescuer will perform the jaw thrust while the other delivers the oxygen (AHA, 2016). If this maneuver does not open the airway, you can switch to the head tilt–chin lift if the airway is obstructed.

First, stand directly behind the child's's head and place your elbows on the area behind the victim's head so that your hands can comfortably reach the jaw area (AHA, 2016). Next, "Place your fingers under the angles of the victim's lower jaw and lift with both hands, displacing the jaw forward" (AHA, 2016, p. 22). This allows you to relieve an obstruction and open the airway. See Image 6 for the correct technique. It is important to ensure the child's mouth does not close, and if it does, position the mouth open by pressing the chin downward (AHA, 2016).

Pediatric Rescue Breathing

If, as a rescuer, you determine the pediatric victim has a pulse present but abnormal breathing, rescue breathing is appropriate. It is important to differentiate abnormal breathing from agonal gasps because agonal gasps can signal impending cardiac arrest; furthermore, presence of agonal gasps should prompt you to begin cardiopulmonary resuscitation (AHA, 2016). The two oxygen delivery devices that are primarily used in adult BLS are also used in pediatric BLS. They are a pocket mask and bag-valve mask.

Device 1 – Pocket Mask

Pocket masks have replaced face shields because they're associated with decreased rates of infection transmission (AHA, 2016). This type of mask is available for civilians to purchase in case of emergency. They can also be found in all medical settings that are equipped with first aid gear (see Image 7).

The pocket mask comes in different sizes to accommodate adult, pediatric, and infant victims. Most pocket masks are equipped with a one-way valve that ensures fluid expelled from the victim is not directed toward the rescuer (AHA, 2016). This valve changes the direction of the victim's expiratory air and all secretions or vomit (AHA, 2016). The top of the mask has an opening that allows you to breathe into the mask for oxygen delivery. It is important to familiarize yourself with this device and become comfortable placing it on a victim's face.

To correctly place a pocket mask, kneel or stand to the side of the child. The "pointy" end of the pocket mask fits over the child's nose with the wide part below the mouth. The mask should be pressed firmly against the child's face so that a seal is created. This seal can be made using the following method:

1. Use the index finger and thumb on the hand that is closest to the top of the child to form a "C" shape around the air inlet. Your fingers should create a seal that prevents air leakage around the nose.
2. Use the thumb of your opposite hand to compress the lower portion of the face mask to the child's face. Use the fingers from the same hand to open the airway by lifting the jaw and completing a head tilt–chin lift.
3. Lower yourself to the pocket mask and breathe into the mask. It will take 1 second to deliver an effective breath.
4. You will know if your oxygen delivery was effective if you see the child's chest rise with each delivered breath (AHA, 2016).

Device 2 – Bag Valve Mask

Another device frequently used by medical professionals during pediatric BLS is a bag-valve mask. A BVM delivers ample oxygen to pediatric victims who are apneic or breathing abnormally. This device can be used while attached to oxygen or without supplemental oxygen. If used with oxygen, the BVM will deliver 100% oxygen; without an oxygen supply, the BVM delivers 21% oxygen, which is the amount of oxygen present in the air (AHA, 2016). The name denotes exactly what the device comprises: a bag, a valve, and a mask. The bag is usually self-inflating, and the valve is non-rebreathing. This means the child receives the appropriate amount of oxygenation and does not inhale carbon dioxide. This mask differs from the pocket mask because it has more cushion and ability to provide a snug fit around the nose and mouth. This design prevents air leakage. Both masks and bags vary in size to fit adults, children, and infants (see Image 17).

It is important to locate the oxygen inlet on the opposite end of the mask to connect oxygen supply when needed. Another key part of the BVM is the reservoir bag (as seen in Image 8). This bag allows for high concentrations of oxygen to be maintained with BVM use; each time the bag is compressed, it fills with highly concentrated oxygen instead of room air containing 21% oxygen (AHA, 2016).

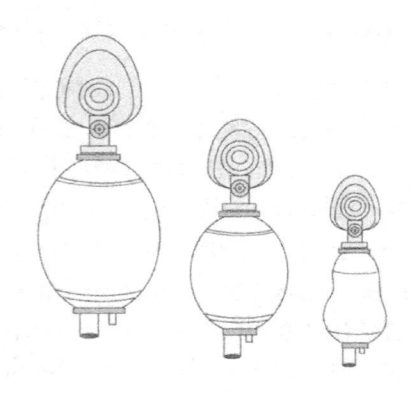

Image 17.

Proper use of the BVM begins with positioning. Begin by standing or kneeling above the victim's head. Next, use the E-C method to ensure a tight seal around the victim's nose and mouth. This technique is best performed with two rescuers, but it can be performed with one as well. Steps for single-rescuer BVM use include:

1. Place the mask on the child's face with the "pointy" end over the nose and the wider portion below the mouth. Pull the bag toward the side you will be compressing while ensuring the bag is perpendicular to the child's body. Keep the bag level so that the air supply is not cut off.
2. Form a "C" shape with your thumb and index finger and wrap this around the mask, keeping close to the edge of the mask.
3. Form an "E" with your middle, ring, and pinky fingers, and lift the jaw upward. This mimics a head tilt–chin lift.
4. While ensuring a tight seal with one hand, use the other hand to compress the bag. It is unnecessary to forcefully squeeze the bag, as this can cause increased intrathoracic pressure over time.

5. A slow, steady squeeze will deliver an effective breath. You will know if your oxygen delivery was effective if you see the child's chest rise with each bag compression (AHA, 2016).

2-rescuer BVM use is the preferred method because the child will receive higher quality ventilation. While your partner uses both hands to ensure the mask is completely sealed while you compress the bag to deliver the breath, or vice versa. More detailed steps include:

1. Your partner will stand above the victim's head and position the mask over the victim's face while you stand to the side of the victim.
2. Using the aforementioned "EC" method, your partner seals the mask to the victim's face on one side and then mirrors this technique on the other side. This ensures a complete, circumferential seal.
3. You can now squeeze the bag to deliver a breath at a slow, steady rate.

Unavailable Equipment

If equipment is unavailable for the provision of airway support (e.g., pocket mask or BVM), there are other practices that can be implemented to provide breaths. Although these practices increase the risk for disease or infection transmission, they can be life-saving interventions for some. The AHA encourages hands-only cardiopulmonary resuscitation (CPR) if airway equipment is unavailable (2020); however, this should be modified to include breaths for children because precipitating factors for pediatric BLS frequently induce hypoxemia, or low blood oxygen level (AHA, 2016). In other words, providing breaths for pediatric victims is imperative because they have a smaller blood oxygen reservoir than adult victims.

In this case, mouth-to-mouth breathing is appropriate for children. Here is how to properly deliver breaths when equipment is unavailable:

1. Perform a head tilt–chin lift.
2. Use your index finger and thumb to close the victim's nose (AHA, 2016).
3. Make a seal with your mouth and provide one breath until you see the victim's chest rise (AHA, 2016).

Scenario

As a daycare worker, you decide to take a group of preschool-aged children outside to play since the weather is nice. You notice a few children standing around a classmate who is lying on the ground. What will you do next?

Action

After you **verify environmental safety**, **complete an initial assessment**, and **shout for help/initiate emergency response system contact**, you palpate a strong carotid pulse on the child. However, the child is breathing abnormally (not gasping). Another daycare worker promptly arrives with emergency equipment, including a pocket mask. You place the pocket mask on the child's face, ensure a tight seal, **complete a head tilt–chin lift**, and give the child rescue breaths. While performing child rescue breaths, you remember the following:

- Give 1 rescue breath every 3-5 seconds. This will total 12-20 breaths every minute (AHA, 2016).
- Signs of poor perfusion (e.g., weak pulse, paleness, mottling, and cyanosis) accompanied with bradycardia (heart rate less than 60 beats per minute) indicate

impending cardiac arrest and warrant the start of chest compressions (AHA, 2016).
- For pediatric BLS, delivering breaths must always be performed if chest compressions are initiated. This is because precipitating factors for pediatric BLS frequently induce hypoxemia, or low blood oxygen level (AHA, 2016).

CHAPTER 8:
AUTOMATED EXTERNAL DEFIBRILLATOR

An automated external defibrillator is a small, portable machine that is found in various locations such as a hospital, school, factory, home, or store (Mayo Clinic, 2020). This machine provides unsynchronized electrical shock to rhythms identified as shockable, such as ventricular fibrillation or pulseless ventricular tachycardia (AHA, 2016; Zoll, n.d.). If the rhythm is not shockable, the AED will advise you to continue chest compressions without defibrillation (Mayo Clinic, 2020). Examples of non-shockable rhythms include pulseless electrical activity and asystole.

Early defibrillation is the *best* chance at stopping the leading fatal rhythm encountered during BLS—ventricular fibrillation. Compressions alone are usually not effective in stopping VF (Gu & Chun-Sheng, 2016). The Mayo Clinic stresses the importance of early defibrillation and alludes to the brain and organ damage that can result from delayed defibrillation (2020). Therefore, as soon as the AED arrives at the scene, you should attach the electrodes to the victim and begin analyzing the victim's heart rhythm. There are a few differences in AED use for children compared to adults.

Equipment

- An AED equipped with a pediatric dose attenuator allows you to deliver a shock that automatically adjusts for a pediatric victim. This decreases the energy level by 67% (AHA, 2016).
- An AED equipped with pediatric pads and cables also automatically adjusts the energy level for a child victim (see Image 18).

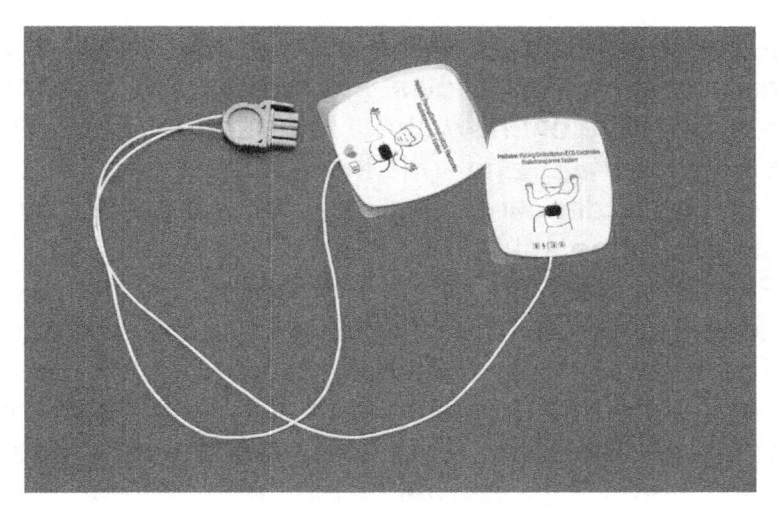

Image 18.

Placement

- If pediatric pads are available, look on the pads themselves for directions. Many pediatric AED pads instruct you to place one pad on the front and one on the back as seen in Image 18. This is referred to as anteroposterior (AP) pad placement (AHA, 2016).
- If only adult pads are available, look on the pads themselves for directions. *It is safe to use adult pads on a child victim.* Although it will provide a stronger shock, "a higher shock dose is preferred to no shock" (AHA, 2016, p. 58).
- If using adult AED pads on a child victim, it is crucial that the pads stay independent of one another to prevent safety issues or hindering shock capability (AHA, 2016).
- According to AHA (2016), child victims over the age of 8 require adult pads because pediatric pads will not provide ample energy.

The precise steps involved in AED use include:

1. Place the AED beside the child on the opposite side of the compressor. This allows you or a partner to complete your resuscitative efforts without interruption (AHA, 2016).
2. Open the AED and turn the machine on. Often, the AED will begin directing you through audible prompts. Listen closely to the steps.
3. Peel the backing off the provided electrodes/pads and adhere them to the child's skin in the correct locations. There should be a visual diagram in the AED pack to ensure correct placement. If you only have adult pads, check to see if the AED is equipped with a pediatric dose attenuator. This special equipment decreases the energy level that reaches the child victim's heart. There are different locations for AED pad placement; therefore, you must look at the pads themselves for direction. Don't forget the main principle of pad placement: the heart must be in-between the pads because electric shock moves between them. Depending on the pad's directions, the pads could be placed on the chest and back in an AP fashion (see Image 18).
4. Plug the electrodes into the AED and wait for the next prompt from the machine. It will direct you to stop compressions for a momentary analysis of the victim's heart rhythm. It is extremely important to stop compressions at this time to ensure proper heart rhythm analysis.
5. If the child's heart rhythm is deemed shockable, the AED will prompt you to take all hands off the child. A common term for this step is to "clear" the victim (AHA, 2016).

    a. Recent evidence suggests that there are benefits to completing compressions in between heart rhythm analysis and shock. This optimizes coronary perfusion and increases the chance for survival (AHA, 2016).

6. Ensure everyone is clear of the victim (including the person delivering breaths) before pressing the shock button.
7. Once you press the shock button, the compressor should immediately resume chest compressions. It may be tempting to palpate for a pulse before starting chest compressions, but this will hinder resuscitation efforts. It is more effective to continue chest compressions.
8. The AED will continue to work and advise you to re-analyze the heart rhythm after two minutes have elapsed. Continue to provide chest compressions in between rhythm analysis. This increases the victim's chance of survival (AHA, 2016).

Here is a simplified version of AED use:

1. Turn on the AED machine.
2. Attach the AED's electrodes to the child's skin in the correct locations.
3. Plug the electrodes into the AED machine.
4. Press the analyze button to determine if the rhythm is shockable.
5. Direct all rescuers to remove their hands from the child.
6. Press the shock button if the rhythm is shockable.
7. Immediately restart chest compressions.

Exceptional Conditions

Under certain conditions, there may be additional considerations that you should take prior to using an AED. Therefore, it's important to pay attention to each unique victim and assess the situation for possible obstacles. When removing a victim's clothing to expose the chest for placement of AED electrodes, you should note whether the victim is wearing any patches or has any implanted devices.

Medication patches that are adhered to the victim's skin can impede an AED's electrical shock. In addition, AED electrodes placed on top of them can produce minor burns. Medication patches must be removed prior to placement of AED pads to avoid these consequences. Before removing the patch, however, don gloves to ensure the medication is not transferred to your skin with removal. Once you have gloves on, take the medication patch off and wipe the area to remove any remaining medication. The patch should be placed in a sharps container to prevent accidental exposure to others or the environment.

Implanted cardiac defibrillators and pacemakers are usually easy to detect because of their prominent figure. For adults, the most common location is the upper chest (see Image 10), but this may vary for children. If an AED electrode is placed over one of these devices, electrical shock will be prevented from reaching the heart. Therefore, you must place the electrodes to the side, above, or below the device to ensure proper energy delivery. It is critical to place the electrodes so that the victim's heart is in between the pads. This allows for electrical conduction to reach the heart.

CHAPTER 9:
PERFORMING SINGLE-RESCUER PEDIATRIC BASIC LIFE SUPPORT

Let's gather the individual tools of BLS and learn how to perform Single-Rescuer Pediatric BLS. Before we begin, let's review the main concepts of BLS for children:

1. Ensuring environmental safety
2. Performing an initial assessment
3. Contacting the emergency response system

    a. In pediatric BLS, you may need to modify and/or merge the step to contact the emergency response system and the 10-second check step depending on whether the collapse was witnessed.

4. Completing a 10-second check
5. Performing chest compressions
6. Managing the victim's airway
7. Using the AED

Scenario

It's a snowy Saturday and you decide to take your 5-year-old nephew sledding in a local field. After going down the hill a few times, your nephew collapses to the ground. You think he is playing a game with you, but you quickly realize he needs emergency care. What will you do?

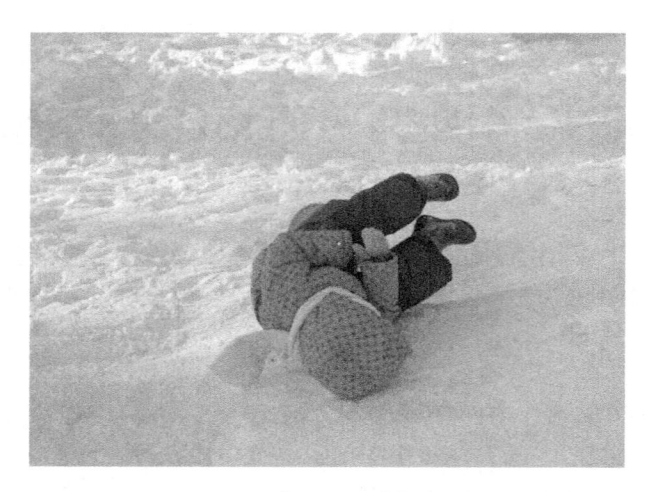

Image 19.

Action

It is time to apply your knowledge of pediatric BLS and act! First, **inspect the environment to ensure the safety** of yourself and the victim. If there were multiple sledders and the child were in the pathway of the sleds, moving the victim to safety would be necessary. However, there are no other sledders or people around. It is important to remember that AED use is safe when the victim is lying on snow, so this would not be a reason to move the victim.

After confirming environmental safety, it's time to **perform an initial assessment** of the victim. Place your hand on the child's shoulder. Simultaneously shake the shoulder and shout to see if the victim responds. Examples of what to shout include "Are you there?" or "Can you open your eyes?" The AVPU tool can further help classify the victim's LOC. While completing this initial assessment, you quickly scan the victim's body for any other obvious injury, but you see nothing abnormal.

This victim remains unresponsive to your attempts at awakening or eliciting a response. Therefore, you begin to **yell for help**. You see no one else in sight, so you quickly perform a **10-second**

check. You place two fingers on the child's carotid artery. You are careful to not use your thumb because of the potential for feeling your own pulse. As you are palpating for the presence of a pulse, you closely watch the victim's chest for any sign of inspiration or expiration. You determine, within 10 seconds, that he does not have a palpable pulse and is not breathing.

Because you witnessed the child's collapse and have determined pulselessness and apnea, you immediately run to the gas station across the street to retrieve an AED. While retrieving the AED in the gas station, you shout for someone to call 9-1-1. You begin running back to the child.

As soon as you return to the child, you quickly open the device and turn on the machine. While it is powering on, you tear the child's shirt away to prepare for pad placement. The device prompts you to place the pads on the victim's skin. The AED is not equipped with pediatric pads, so you place the first adult pad on the child's chest and the second adult pad on the child's back. You ensure the pads are independent of one another and not touching.

As the AED analyzes the victim's rhythm, you remain clear of the victim. Shock is advised, so you start chest compressions until it is time to press the shock button. Before pressing the button, you make sure you are not touching the victim. Immediately after pressing the shock button, you restart quality chest compressions.

For quality **chest compressions**, you place one heel of the hand on the lower part of the breastbone and interlock the other hand on top. While keeping your arms straight and leaning over the child's body, you compress at a rate of 100-120 compressions per minute. You hum the tune of "Stayin' Alive" to keep pace. You compress at least 2 inches or 1/3 the child's chest diameter. The AED has a pocket mask, so you deliver two rescue breaths after 30 compressions. You know that it's especially important to avoid low blood oxygen levels in children.

After two minutes pass, the AED begins analyzing the child's heart rhythm and detects a shockable rhythm. As the unit is charging, you continue compressions but stop when unit is charged. You remain clear of the victim and press the shock button. You immediately resume chest compressions and notice the child begin to move underneath you. You stop compressions and palpate for a carotid pulse. A weak, but present, pulse is palpable! You hear the sirens of the ambulance approaching, so you continue to provide support until the crew arrives.

CHAPTER 10:
PERFORMING 2-RESCUER PEDIATRIC BASIC LIFE SUPPORT

Now, let's assess a different scenario and discuss the appropriate actions when 2 rescuers are available to provide BLS. Before we begin, let's review the main concepts of pediatric BLS one more time:

1. Ensuring environmental safety
2. Performing an initial assessment
3. Contacting the emergency response system

    a. In pediatric BLS, you may need to modify and/or merge the step to contact the emergency response system and the 10-second check step depending on whether the collapse was witnessed.

4. Completing a 10-second check
5. Performing chest compressions
6. Managing the victim's airway
7. Using the AED

Scenario

You are on vacation and relaxing at the hotel pool with your best friend. You see a mother putting sunscreen on her child, who is around 8 years old. Suddenly, the child collapses to the ground and the mother screams for help. What will you do first?

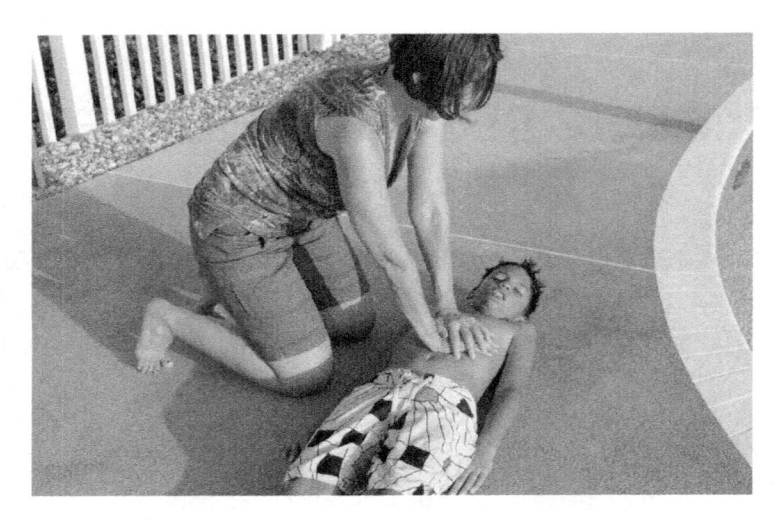

Image 20.

Action

Before approaching the child, it is crucial to **verify environmental safety**. For example, an impending storm with active lightning may necessitate moving the child and yourself to a safe location. Also, a large amount of water underneath the child could compromise your safety due to electrical conduction if an AED is used. The surface under the child is damp, so no movement is necessary.

Your friend **begins the initial assessment** by shaking the child's shoulder and shouting, "Are you there?" No response from the child indicates unresponsiveness and warrants contacting the emergency response system. You direct your friend to call 9-1-1 and retrieve an AED.

You place two fingers between the child's trachea and neck muscles to determine for the presence of a carotid pulse (AHA, 2016). This is **completed in 10 seconds** while scanning the victim's chest for inspiration or expiration. Assessment reveals pulselessness and apnea.

You immediately **begin chest compressions**. The child is in swimming trunks, so the clothes do not need to be moved aside because the chest is exposed. You compress at a rate of 100-120 compressions per minute at a depth of at least 2 inches (or 1/3 the diameter of the child's chest). The heel of one hand is on the lower part of the child's breastbone with the other hand interlocked. Ensuring your arms are straight and body leaned over the child's body, the victim's chest re-expands between each compression for optimal cardiac perfusion. You recognize the surface underneath the victim (concrete patio) is appropriate resistance for chest compressions. You do not have a pocket mask available, so you continue providing continuous compressions.

Your friend arrives with emergency equipment, including an AED and pocket mask. Therefore, your friend starts attaching the AED pads while you continue to provide compressions. Your friend turns the device on, and it begins analyzing the child's heart rhythm. You take your hands off the child for heart rhythm analysis. The AED determines the child does not have a shockable heart rhythm. So, you continue chest compressions and your friend provides airway support in sets of 15 compressions and 2 breaths. After two minutes, the AED analyzes the child's heart rhythm again. The rhythm is still not shockable, so you switch roles with your friend and continue providing sets of 15 compressions and 2 breaths.

Your friend states, "He just moved!" So, you quickly assess for the presence of a carotid pulse while your friend pauses chest compressions. You palpate a weak, but present, carotid pulse! The child begins to groan, and you provide supportive care as the emergency response team approaches the scene.

UNIT 3:
INFANT BASIC LIFE SUPPORT

Although infant cardiopulmonary arrest is a frightening event, parents, caregivers, bystanders, and medical personnel must be prepared to act. Infant BLS is quite different from pediatric and adult BLS, and knowledge of these differences is pivotal to victim survival. Let's discuss these differences and become confident in our ability to provide resuscitation to infants in distress.

CHAPTER 11:
FUNDAMENTALS

Infant, child, and adult BLS share a common goal: restore normal heart and respiratory function. O'Connor states that 50-65% of children who suffer cardiac arrest and require BLS are under the age of 1 year (2019). This staggering statistic underscores the importance of understanding the technique of infant BLS. Infant BLS applies to victims under the age of 1 year old and does not apply to newborns (AHA, 2016). Let's learn the fundamentals of infant BLS, including environmental safety, initial assessment, emergency response system contact, 10-second check, and chest compressions.

Environmental Safety

Like adult and child BLS, the first step in infant BLS is confirming environmental safety. This safety check provides crucial information about the scene and prevents undue harm to you or other rescuers (AHA, 2016). The American Red Cross recommends carefully inspecting the environment for potential hazards, including toxic debris, rapid water, smoke, traffic, live electrical wires, unsteady structures, or severe weather (2011). If the environment is deemed hazardous, then you should seek safety and alert emergency personnel of an identified victim and their location (ARC, 2011). If the environment is deemed safe, you should approach the victim while maintaining situational awareness.

There are certain situations that necessitate moving an infant to a safe place before performing BLS. For example, an infant who is lying in a large puddle of water will need to be moved to a dry location because BLS often involves the use of an AED. Furthermore, using an AED while the infant is in water could cause harm to rescuers because of electrical conduction (University of

Missouri, n.d.). A victim on snow or in a small amount of water does not need to be moved prior to AED use; however, water droplets present on the victim's chest need to be dried (AHA, 2016).

In addition to environmental safety, you must ensure personal safety by donning the correct personal protective equipment before touching any bodily fluids. This prevents unnecessary exposure and potential transmission of blood-borne illnesses.

While donning the appropriate PPE, you can quickly inspect the victim's primary injury or problem. This allows you to prioritize and optimize rescue efforts. For example, you would be demonstrating poor prioritization if you became focused on checking for pupillary response instead of treating the infant's agonal breathing. You must prioritize and treat according to the primary threat to the victim's survival (Thim et al., 2012).

Initial Assessment

After the environment is considered safe or the infant is moved to a safe area, you must perform an initial assessment. This begins with assessing the infant's responsiveness. Consider using this approach:

- Kneel beside the victim.
- Simultaneously tap the infant's heel and shout to awaken (AHA, 2016).

After the infant's responsiveness is established, you can proceed based on immediate need. For the purposes of this guide, we will assume the infant is unresponsive and requires BLS.

Emergency Response System Contact

A lone rescuer needs assistance in an emergency. This is true for hospital or non-hospital settings. You should shout for help in either setting. When assistance arrives, you should direct that person to retrieve emergency equipment, such as an AED.

One key difference between adult and child/infant BLS is the correct time to retrieve the AED if no assistance is available. To review, in adult BLS, you should immediately retrieve the AED if the victim is deemed unresponsive and you are unable to activate the emergency response system (e.g., no cell phone). In infant BLS, however, you must base your actions on whether the collapse was witnessed. If the collapse was witnessed and the infant is unresponsive or pulseless (complete the 10-second check), leave the scene to immediately get the AED and initiate emergency response system contact (AHA, 2016). If the collapse was not witnessed and the child or infant is unresponsive or pulseless (complete the 10-second check), you should complete sets of 30 chest compressions and 2 breaths for two minutes before leaving the scene to retrieve the AED and initiate contact with the emergency response system (AHA, 2016). To summarize, *in infant BLS, you may need to merge the step to contact the emergency response system contact and the 10-second check step depending on whether the collapse was witnessed.* Let's reiterate these key points:

- Witnessed collapse → If alone, leave to get the AED and initiate contact.
- Unwitnessed collapse → If alone, complete two minutes of chest compressions before leaving to get the AED and initiate contact.

Technology can be very useful in BLS scenarios because of hands-free options. When initiating contact with the emergency response system (e.g., dialing 9-1-1), it is paramount to place the device on speakerphone to allow freedom of both hands for continued resuscitation efforts.

If in a hospital setting, shout for nearby help or activate the hospital's emergency response system (e.g., press the code blue button). Often, the hospital's phone system has a specific code that can be entered to override the phone system and notify the operator of an emergency. When speaking with the operator, it is crucial to give the victim's location and type of emergency assistance needed. For example, you can tell the operator, "Code Blue, NICU, room 4." This will initiate the hospital's emergency response team, which often includes designated team members from anesthesia, critical care (provider and registered nurses), respiratory therapy, and laboratory. If the victim is experiencing an acute stroke, radiology will be called to attend the code. Predesignated, experienced code teams allow for smooth assessment and immediate intervention. Without code team designation, a rush of responders would cause chaos, incite confusion, and hamper resuscitation efforts.

Healthcare workers must become familiar with their institution's emergency procedures and protocols. This optimizes patient safety and emergency responses. A color-coded chart may be offered at some institutions (see Image 3). These are often required to be placed within sight or on an employee's badge. Different colors designate the emergency and signal specific personnel to respond.

10-Second Check

The next critical step merges two assessments: pulse and breathing. Conducting these assessments simultaneously enables you to begin BLS without delay. *In infant BLS, you may need to merge the step to contact the emergency response system contact and the 10-second check step depending on whether the collapse was witnessed.* For an infant victim, place two fingers on the infant's brachial artery (inner upper arm) while watching for inspiration or expiration. If unable to palpate the brachial pulse, it is appropriate to assess for a femoral pulse. Avoid using the thumb as this can cause you to mistakenly palpate your own pulse. See Image 21 for reference. In total, assessing the infant's breathing and pulse should be completed within 10 seconds (AHA, 2016). This step is often referred to as "Look, listen, and feel" (Schlesinger, 2011).

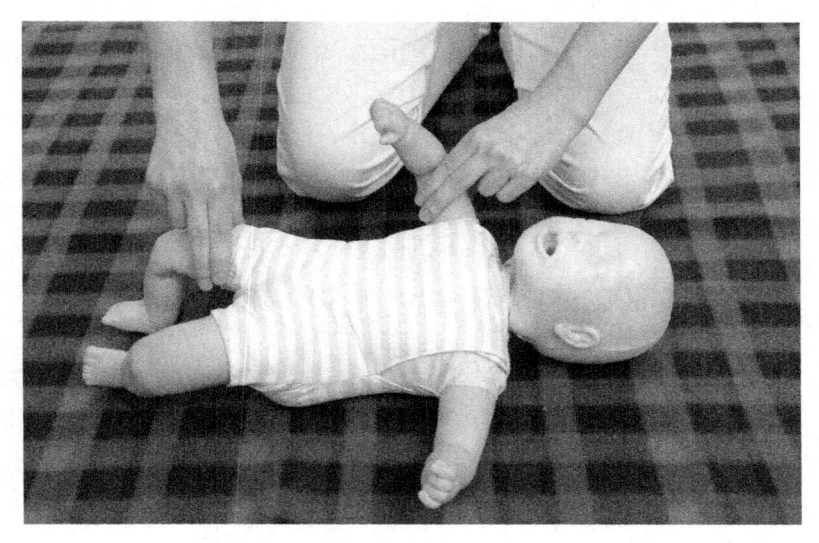

Image 21.

If the infant is determined to be pulseless and is not breathing, CPR should be initiated immediately. If the infant has a pulse but abnormal breathing, you should initiate rescue breathing. If the infant has a pulse and is breathing normally, remain beside the infant and provide support until emergency help arrives (AHA, 2016).

Chest Compressions

One component of BLS stands out as the single most important part of resuscitation—chest compressions. Simply put, chest compressions pump blood to the brain and other vital organs, and survival is *directly* linked with compression quality. Poor compression quality is called "a preventable harm" and can decrease the rate of survival rate by as much as 30% (Meaney et al., 2013, p. 418).

For an infant victim, follow these steps:

- Kneel or stand beside the victim depending on whether the infant is on the ground or in a bed/crib.
- *Optional:* Remove the infant's clothing to allow for proper inspection of anatomical locations (for example, the breastbone) and prepare for AED arrival.
- For single-rescuer infant BLS chest compressions, compress in the middle of the infant's chest on the lower part of the breastbone. It is important to avoid compressing on the end of the breastbone (AHA, 2016). See Image 22.
- For 2-rescuer infant BLS chest compressions, wrap your hands around the infant so that your fingertips are resting on the infant's lower back. Then, using both thumbs, compress in the middle of the infant's chest. This is called the *encircling hands technique* (AHA, 2016). See Image 23.
- You should compress the infant's chest "at least one third the AP diameter of the infant' chest (about 1.5 inches [4cm])" (AHA, 2016, p. 50).
- Complete at least 100-120 compressions per minute. To keep pace, compress to the tune of "Stayin' Alive" by the Bee Gees (AHA, 2020).
- Stay committed to continual compressions and avoid interruptions. This keeps blood flowing through the heart and to the rest of the body. Any interruption interferes with the infant's survival.
- Ensure the chest re-expands or recoils completely between each compression. Without full expansion, the heart and brain are not perfused properly and the infant's mean arterial pressure (MAP) declines (Yannopoulos et al., 2005).

- Ensure the infant is on a firm surface. A soft surface will absorb the compression effort and render the compressions ineffective. A firm surface opposes the compression force, thereby allowing a complete compression and perfusion (AHA, 2016).
- In an ideal situation, there should be at least 2 rescuers, and you should switch every two minutes. Providing chest compressions is very tiring, and rest periods are crucial for rescuers to provide quality compressions (AHA, 2016).

Here is a simplified version:

- Kneel or stand beside the infant.
- Compress in the middle of the infant's chest using 2 fingers if alone.
- If another rescuer is present, use the encircling hands technique, compressing with both thumbs.
- Complete 100-120 compressions per minute.
- Allow full chest expansion between compressions.
- Do not stop until AED arrival.

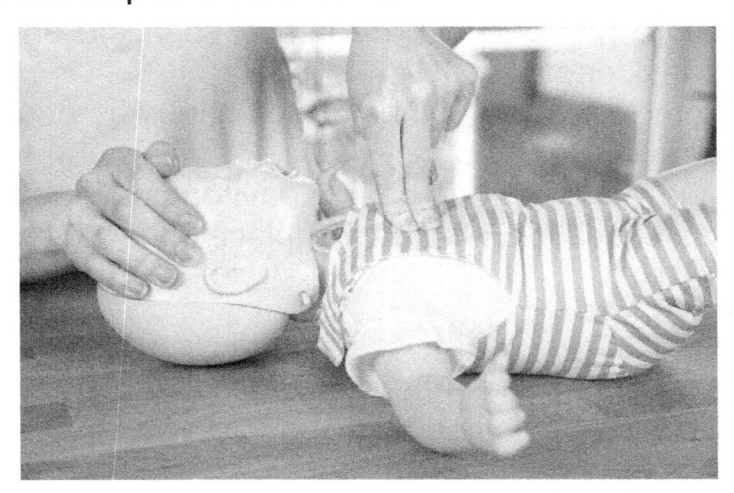

Image 22.

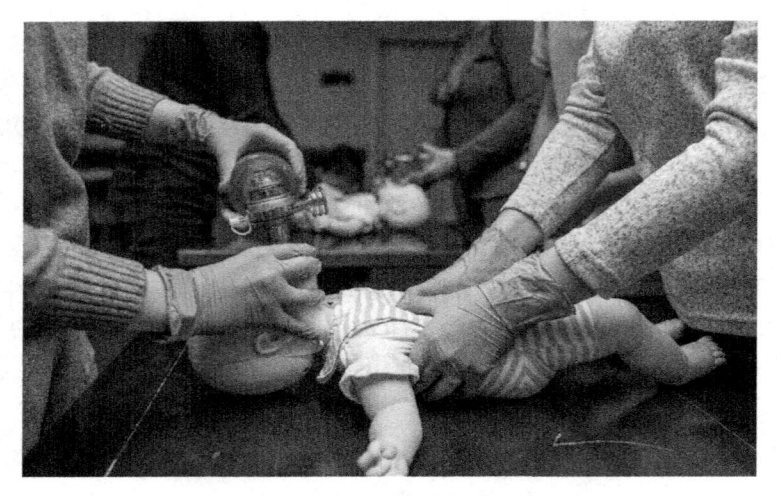

Image 23.

Infant BLS Fundamentals Review

Let's review what we just learned and select three key points from each section to commit to memory.

Environmental safety

1. Before approaching the infant, scan the environment for safety concerns.
2. Protect yourself from injury or illness by donning the correct PPE.
3. If the victim is in an unsafe environment, move the child to a safe location if it does not place either of you in danger.

Initial assessment

1. Assess the child's responsiveness.
2. Tap the infant's heel and shout to awaken.

Emergency response system contact

1. Regardless of setting, shout for help.

2. Use speakerphone to dial 9-1-1.
3. In infant BLS, you may need to modify and/or merge the step to contact the emergency response system and the 10-second check step depending on whether the collapse was witnessed.

    a. Witnessed collapse → If alone, leave to get the AED and initiate contact.
    b. Unwitnessed collapse → If alone, complete two minutes of chest compressions before leaving to get the AED and initiate contact.

10-second check

1. Place two fingers on the infant's brachial or femoral artery.
2. Watch chest for expiration or inspiration during pulse check.
3. Complete these steps simultaneously within 10 seconds.

Chest compressions

1. Ensure the victim is on a firm surface.
2. Use 2 fingers in the middle of the infant's chest to compress during single-rescuer infant BLS.
3. Use the encircling hands technique, compressing with your thumbs, during 2-rescuer infant BLS (AHA, 2016).
4. Compress at least 1.5 inches (or 1/3 the AP diameter of the chest) at a rate of 100-120 compressions/minute while allowing chest re-expansion between each compression (AHA, 2016).

CHAPTER 12:
AIRWAY MANAGEMENT

The airway can be challenging to manage because every victim's anatomy is slightly different. Whether an adult, child, or infant victim, the first goal in airway management during BLS is to open the airway. There are two maneuvers that facilitate airway opening and allow for oxygen delivery.

Maneuver 1 – Head tilt–chin lift

The first maneuver is the most performed airway technique for an unresponsive infant. It is called the *head tilt–chin lift* and should only be performed on an infant who *does not* have a potential neck or head injury (AHA, 2016). After placing one hand on the victim's forehead, apply pressure to tilt the victim's head toward the ground. In infants, tilting the head back too far may obstruct the airway because of their anatomical prematurity. It is critical to not tilt the head "beyond the neutral (sniffing) position" (AHA, 2016, p. 52). Following this guideline ensures airway patency and proper positioning for oxygen delivery.

Next, take your other hand and position your fingers underneath the infant's chin. Lastly, pull the chin upward to open the airway and shift the tongue out of the way (AHA, 2016). Avoid pressing into the soft tissue at the anterior of the neck (AHA, 2016). This could create further oxygenation issues and hamper obstruction relief attempts. See Image 24 to see how to properly perform the head tilt–chin lift technique on an infant victim.

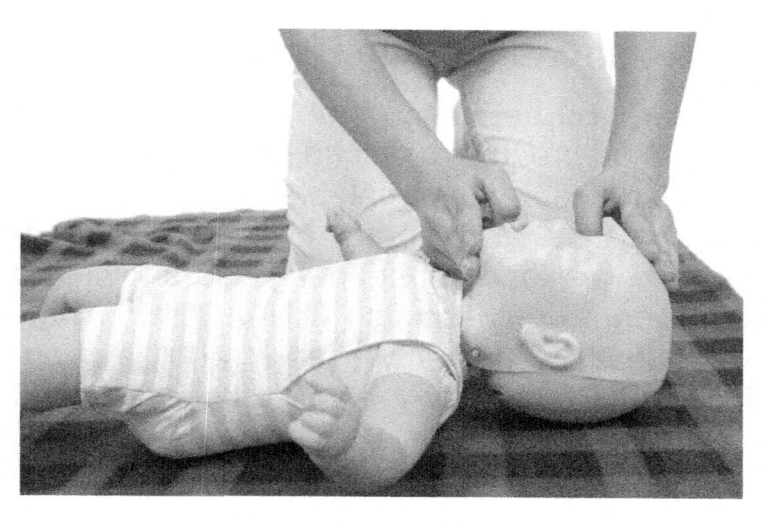

Image 24.

Maneuver 2 – Jaw Thrust

As with adult and child BLS, the second maneuver that can be implemented for infants with airway issues (and victims with potential head or neck injuries) is the jaw thrust. For an infant, this maneuver takes moderate strength and two hands to complete; therefore, one rescuer will perform the jaw thrust while the other delivers the oxygen (AHA, 2016). If this maneuver does not open the airway, you can switch to the head tilt–chin lift if the airway is obstructed.

To perform a jaw thrust, stand directly behind the infant's head and place your elbows on the area behind the infant's head so that the hands can comfortably reach the jaw area (AHA, 2016). Next, "Place your fingers under the angles of the victim's lower jaw and lift with both hands, displacing the jaw forward" (AHA, 2016, p. 22). This allows you to relieve an obstruction and open the airway. It is important to ensure the infant's mouth does not close, and if it does, position the mouth open by pressing the chin downward (AHA, 2016).

Infant Rescue Breathing

If, as a rescuer, you determine that an infant victim has a pulse present but abnormal breathing, rescue breathing is appropriate. It is important to differentiate abnormal breathing from agonal gasps because agonal gasps accompany or signal impending cardiac arrest; furthermore, presence of agonal gasps should prompt you to begin cardiopulmonary resuscitation (AHA, 2016). The two oxygen delivery devices that are primarily used in adult and child BLS are also used in infant BLS. They are a pocket mask and bag-valve mask.

Device 1 – Pocket Mask

Pocket masks have replaced face shields because they're associated with decreased rates of infection transmission (AHA, 2016). This type of mask is available for civilians to purchase in case of emergency. They can also be found in all medical settings that are equipped with first aid gear (see Image 7).

The pocket mask comes in different sizes to accommodate adult, child, and infant victims. Most pocket masks are equipped with a one-way valve that ensures fluid expelled from the victim is not directed toward the rescuer (AHA, 2016). This valve changes the direction of the victim's expiratory air and all secretions or vomit (AHA, 2016). The top of the mask has an opening that allows you to breathe into the mask for oxygen delivery. It is important to familiarize yourself with this device and become comfortable placing it on an infant's face. A properly fitting pocket mask will not cover the infant's eyes or extend beyond the chin; instead, it should only cover the infant's mouth and nose (AHA, 2016).

To correctly place a pocket mask, kneel or stand to the side of the infant. The "pointy" end of the pocket mask fits over the infant's nose with the wide part below the mouth. The mask should be pressed firmly against the infant's face so that a seal is created. This seal can be made using the following method:

1. Use the index finger and thumb on the hand that is closest to the top of the infant to form a "C" shape around the air inlet. Your fingers should create a seal that prevents air leakage around the nose.
2. Use the thumb of your opposite hand to compress the lower portion of the face mask to the infant's face. Use the fingers from the same hand to open the airway by lifting the jaw and completing a head tilt–chin lift.
3. Lower yourself to the pocket mask and breathe into the mask. It will take 1 second to deliver an effective breath.
4. You will know if your oxygen delivery was effective if you see the infant's chest rise with each delivered breath (AHA, 2016).

Device 2 – Bag Valve Mask

Another device frequently used by medical professionals during infant BLS is a bag-valve mask. A BVM delivers ample oxygen to infant victims who are apneic or breathing abnormally. This device can be used while attached to oxygen or without supplemental oxygen. If used with oxygen, the BVM will deliver 100% oxygen; without an oxygen supply, the BVM delivers 21% oxygen, which is the amount of oxygen present in the air (AHA, 2016).

The name denotes exactly what the device comprises: a bag, a valve, and a mask. The bag is usually self-inflating, and the valve is non-rebreathing. This means the infant receives the appropriate amount of oxygenation and does not inhale carbon dioxide. This mask differs from the pocket mask because it has more cushion and ability to provide a snug fit around the nose and mouth. This design prevents air leakage. Both masks and bags vary in size to fit adults, children, and infants (see Image 17).

It is important to locate the oxygen inlet on the opposite end of the mask to connect oxygen supply when needed. Another part of the BVM worth discussing is the reservoir bag (as seen in Image 8). This bag allows for the maintenance of highly concentrated oxygen. In other words, each time the bag is compressed, it fills with highly concentrated oxygen instead of room air containing 21% oxygen (AHA, 2016).

Proper use of the BVM begins with positioning. You must stand or kneel above the infant's head. Next, use the "EC" method to ensure a tight seal around the infant's nose and mouth. This technique is best performed with two rescuers, but it can be performed with one as well. Steps for single-rescuer BVM use include:

1. Place the mask on the infant's face with the "pointy" end over the nose and the wider portion below the mouth. Pull the bag toward the side you will be compressing while ensuring the bag is perpendicular to the infant's body. Keep the bag level so that the air supply is not cut off.
2. Form a "C" shape with your thumb and index finger and wrap this around the mask, keeping close to the edge of the mask.
3. Form an "E" with your middle, ring, and pinky fingers, and lift the jaw upward. This mimics a head tilt–chin lift.
4. While ensuring a tight seal with one hand, use the other hand to compress the bag. It is unnecessary to forcefully squeeze the bag, as this can cause increased intrathoracic pressure over time.
5. A slow, steady squeeze will deliver an effective breath. You will know if your oxygen delivery was effective if you see the infant's chest rise with each bag compression (AHA, 2016).

2-rescuer BVM use is the preferred method because the infant will receive higher quality ventilation. While your partner uses both hands to ensure the mask is completely sealed while you compress the bag to deliver the breath, or vice versa. More detailed steps include:

1. Your partner will stand above the victim's head and position the mask over the victim's face while you stand to the side of the victim.
2. Using the aforementioned "EC" method, your partner seals the mask to the victim's face on one side and then mirrors this technique on the other side. This ensures a complete, circumferential seal.
3. You can now squeeze the bag to deliver a breath at a slow, steady rate.

Unavailable Equipment

If equipment is unavailable for the provision of airway support (e.g., pocket mask or BVM), there are other practices that can be implemented to provide breaths. Although these practices increase the risk for disease or infection transmission, they can be life-saving interventions for some. The AHA encourages hands-only cardiopulmonary resuscitation (CPR) if airway equipment is unavailable (2020); however, this should be modified to include breaths for children because precipitating factors for pediatric BLS frequently induce hypoxemia, or low blood oxygen level (AHA, 2016). In other words, providing breaths for infant victims is imperative because they have a smaller blood oxygen reservoir than adult victims.

Mouth-to-mouth and mouth-to-mouth-to-nose breathing are both appropriate for infants (AHA, 2016). Here is how to properly deliver breaths via mouth-to-mouth:

1. Perform a head tilt–chin lift.

2. Use your index finger and thumb to close the victim's nose (AHA, 2016).
3. Make a seal with your mouth and provide one breath until you see the victim's chest rise (AHA, 2016).

Similarly, follow these steps for mouth-to-mouth-to-nose breathing:

1. Perform a head tilt–chin lift.
2. Create an airtight seal by positioning "your mouth over the infant's mouth and nose" and provide one breath until you see the victim's chest or abdomen rise (AHA, 2016).

Scenario

It's a Saturday afternoon, and you are watching your sister's 2-month-old infant while she grocery shops. You place the infant in a swing but quickly notice her face looks blue around the mouth. What will you do next?

Action

After you **verify environmental safety**, take her out of the swing, **complete an initial assessment**, and **shout for help/initiate emergency response system contact**, you palpate a strong brachial pulse. The infant begins to breathe abnormally, but not gasping. Your brother-in-law promptly arrives with a first aid kit, including a pocket mask. You place the pocket mask on the infant's face, ensure a tight seal, **complete a head tilt–chin lift**, and give the infant rescue breaths. The appropriate protocol to follow for infant rescue breathing includes:

- Give 1 rescue breath every 3-5 seconds via the pocket mask. This will total 12-20 breaths per minute (AHA, 2016).

- Signs of poor perfusion (e.g., weak pulse, paleness, mottling, and cyanosis) accompanied with bradycardia (heart rate less than 60 beats per minute) indicate impending cardiac arrest and warrant the start of chest compressions in addition to rescue breathing (AHA, 2016).
- For both infant BLS, delivering breaths must always be performed if chest compressions are initiated. This is because precipitating factors for infant BLS frequently induce hypoxemia, or low blood oxygen level (AHA, 2016).

CHAPTER 13:
AUTOMATED EXTERNAL DEFIBRILLATOR

An automated external defibrillator is a small, portable machine that is found in various locations such as a hospital, school, factory, home, or store (Mayo Clinic, 2020). This machine provides unsynchronized electrical shock to rhythms identified as shockable, such as ventricular fibrillation or pulseless ventricular tachycardia (AHA, 2016; Zoll, n.d.). If the rhythm is not shockable, the AED will advise you to continue chest compressions without defibrillation (Mayo Clinic, 2020). Examples of non-shockable rhythms include pulseless electrical activity and asystole.

Early defibrillation is the *best* chance at stopping the leading fatal rhythm encountered during BLS—ventricular fibrillation. Compressions alone are usually not effective in stopping VF (Gu & Chun-Sheng, 2016). The Mayo Clinic stresses the importance of early defibrillation and alludes to the brain and organ damage that can result from delayed defibrillation (2020). Therefore, as soon as the AED arrives to the scene, you should attach the electrodes to the victim and begin analyzing the infant's heart rhythm. There are a few differences in AED use for infants compared to adults.

Equipment

- An AED equipped with a pediatric dose attenuator allows you to deliver a shock that automatically adjusts for a pediatric victim. This decreases the energy level by 67% (AHA, 2016).
- An AED equipped with pediatric pads and cables automatically adjusts the energy level for a pediatric victim.
- Pediatric pads that are used on children can also be used on infant victims. However, if pediatric pads are not

included in the AED, adult pads can be used as well.

Placement

- If pediatric pads are available, look on the pads themselves for directions. Many pediatric AED pads instruct you to place one pad on the front and one on the back as seen in Image 18. This is referred to as anteroposterior (AP) pad placement and is the most frequent placement for an infant victim due to small body surface area (AHA, 2016).
- If only adult pads are available, look on the pads themselves for directions. *It is safe to use adult pads on an infant victim.* Although it will provide a stronger shock than is necessary, "a higher shock dose is preferred to no shock" (AHA, 2016, p. 58).
- If using adult AED pads on a child victim, it is crucial that the pads stay independent of one another to prevent safety issues or hindering shock capability (AHA, 2016).

The precise steps involved in AED use include:

1. Place the AED beside the infant on the opposite side of the compressor. This allows you or a partner to complete your resuscitative efforts without interruption (AHA, 2016).
2. Open the AED and turn the machine on. Often, the AED will begin directing you through audible prompts. Listen closely to the steps.
3. Peel the backing off the provided electrodes/pads and adhere them to the infant's skin in the correct locations. There should be a visual diagram in the AED pack to ensure correct placement. If you only have adult pads, check to see if the AED is equipped with a pediatric dose attenuator. This special equipment decreases the energy

level that reaches the child victim's heart. You must look at the pads themselves for direction. Don't forget the main principle of pad placement: the heart must be in-between the pads because electric shock moves between them. For infant victims, the most frequent placement for pads is on the chest and back in an AP fashion (AHA, 2016).
4. Plug the electrodes into the AED and wait for the next prompt from the machine. It will direct you to stop compressions for a momentary analysis of the victim's heart rhythm. It is extremely important to stop compressions at this time to ensure proper heart rhythm analysis.
5. If the infant's heart rhythm is deemed shockable, the AED will prompt you to take all hands off the infant. A common term for this step is to "clear" the victim (AHA, 2016).

   a. Recent evidence suggests that there are benefits to completing compressions in between heart rhythm analysis and shock. This optimizes coronary perfusion and increases the chance for survival (AHA, 2016).

6. Ensure everyone is clear of the victim (including the person delivering breaths) before pressing the shock button.
7. Once you press the shock button, the compressor should immediately resume chest compressions. It may be tempting to palpate for a pulse before starting chest compressions, but this will hinder resuscitation efforts. It is more effective to continue chest compressions.
8. The AED will continue to work and advise you to re-analyze the heart rhythm after two minutes have elapsed. Continue to provide chest compressions in between rhythm analysis. This increases the victim's chance of survival (AHA, 2016).

Here is a simplified version of AED use:

1. Turn on the AED machine.
2. Attach the AED's electrodes to the infant's skin in the correct locations.
3. Plug in the electrodes to the AED machine.
4. Press the analyze button to determine if the rhythm is shockable.
5. Direct all rescuers to remove their hands from the infant.
6. Press the shock button if the rhythm is shockable.
7. Immediately restart chest compressions.

Exceptional Conditions

Under certain conditions, there may be additional considerations that you should take prior to using an AED. Therefore, it's important to pay attention to each unique victim and assess the situation for possible obstacles. When removing a victim's clothing to expose the chest for placement of AED electrodes, you should note whether the victim is wearing any patches.

Medication patches that are adhered to the victim's skin can impede an AED's electrical shock. In addition, AED electrodes placed on top of them can produce minor burns. Medication patches must be removed prior to placement of AED pads to avoid these consequences. Before removing the patch, however, don gloves to ensure the medication is not transferred to your skin with removal. Once you have gloves on, take the medication patch off and wipe the area to remove any remaining medication. The patch should be placed in a sharps container to prevent accidental exposure to others or the environment.

CHAPTER 14:
PERFORMING SINGLE-RESCUER INFANT BASIC LIFE SUPPORT

Let's gather the individual tools of infant BLS and learn how to perform Single-Rescuer Infant BLS. Before we begin, let's review the main concepts of infant BLS:

1. Ensuring environmental safety
2. Performing an initial assessment
3. Contacting the emergency response system

    a. In infant BLS, you may need to modify and/or merge the step to contact the emergency response system and the 10-second check step depending on whether the collapse was witnessed.

4. Completing a 10-second check
5. Performing chest compressions
6. Managing the victim's airway
7. Using the AED

Scenario

You are taking a walk on a local trail and hear a distressed mother yelling for help. You begin running toward the call for help and see a woman standing over a stroller containing an infant who appears to be sleeping. The mother exclaims, "She isn't breathing or moving!" What will you do?

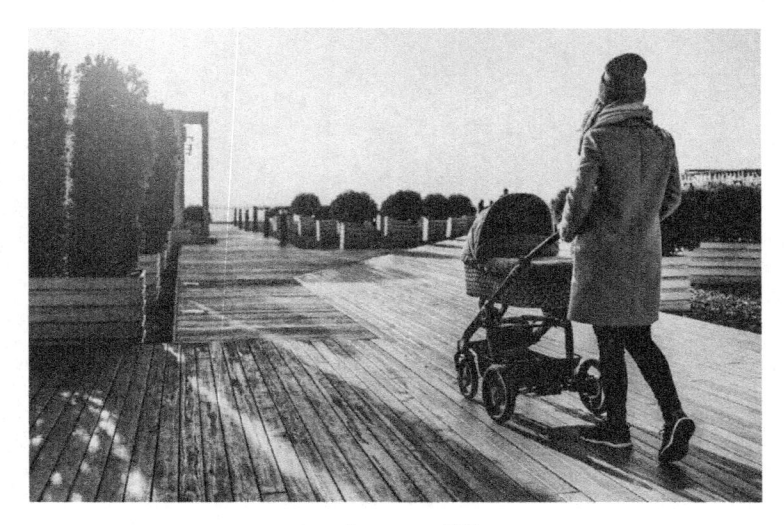

Image 25.

Action

It is time to apply your knowledge of infant BLS and act! First, **inspect the environment to ensure the safety** of yourself and the victim. If the stroller were in the pathway of trail traffic (e.g., bicyclists), it would be necessary to move the stroller aside. It is important to remember that there must be a solid surface underneath a victim requiring chest compressions to ensure adequate perfusion. Therefore, it could also be necessary to move the infant to the ground or pick up the infant to perform BLS. By cradling the infant, you can provide resistance for compressions, deliver rescue breaths, and maintain the mobility to retrieve help if needed. See Image 26 for reference.

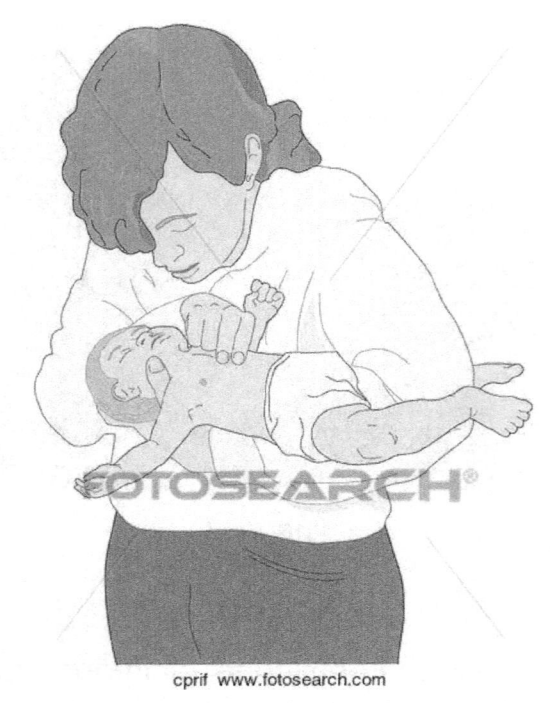

Image 26.

After confirming environmental safety, it is time to **perform an initial assessment** of the victim. Tap or move the infant's heel and shout to determine responsiveness. An example of what to shout is, "Baby, wake up!" The AVPU tool can further help classify the victim's LOC. While completing this initial assessment, you quickly scan the victim's body for any other obvious injury, but you see nothing abnormal.

The infant remains unresponsive to your attempts at awakening or eliciting a response. Therefore, you begin to **yell for help, and instruct the mother to call 9-1-1**. You see no one else in sight, so you quickly perform a **10-second check**. You place two fingers on the infant's brachial artery. You are careful to not use your thumb because of the potential for feeling your own pulse. As you palpate for the presence of a pulse, you closely watch the infant's chest or abdomen for any sign of inspiration or expiration. You determine, within 10 seconds, that she does not have a palpable pulse and is not breathing.

Because you did not witness the precipitating events to the infant's unresponsiveness and have determined pulselessness and apnea, you immediately begin CPR. If the emergency response system is unable to be reached (e.g., no cell phone service), it will be necessary for you to leave the scene to get an AED after two minutes of CPR. Alternatively, you could bring the infant with you and complete CPR while en route.

While completing CPR, you recall the proper technique for single-rescuer infant BLS, which includes placing 2 fingers in the middle of the infant's chest and compressing at least 1.5 inches at a rate of 100-120 compressions per minute.

Fortunately, the mother of the infant is able to reach emergency response personnel and they are expected to arrive within ten minutes. Because you do not have a pocket mask, you weigh the risks versus benefits of completing mouth-to-mouth-to-nose breathing. You decide providing breaths is imperative; therefore, after 30 compressions, you give the infant 2 breaths via mouth-to-mouth-to-nose.

You continue cycles of 30 compressions and 2 breaths for a few more minutes. Soon, the infant begins to move and whimper. You cease CPR and hear the ambulance sirens approaching the scene. The infant has a strong brachial pulse and is becoming more alert! You provide supportive care until the emergency response team arrives.

CHAPTER 15:
PERFORMING 2-RESCUER INFANT BASIC LIFE SUPPORT

Let's assess a different scenario and identify the appropriate actions for 2-rescuer infant BLS. Before we begin, let's review the main concepts of infant BLS:

1. Ensuring environmental safety
2. Performing an initial assessment
3. Contacting the emergency response system

    a. In infant BLS, you may need to modify and/or merge the step to contact the emergency response system and the 10-second check step depending on whether the collapse was witnessed.

4. Completing a 10-second check
5. Performing chest compressions
6. Managing the victim's airway
7. Using the AED

Scenario

You are at the mall with your best friend and her 8-month-old son. Your friend is wearing the infant in a baby carrier as you shop. While walking, you friend begins to panic and shouts because she sees her baby slumped over and unresponsive. You quickly help her take the infant out of the carrier and start to think through performing infant BLS. What is your next step?

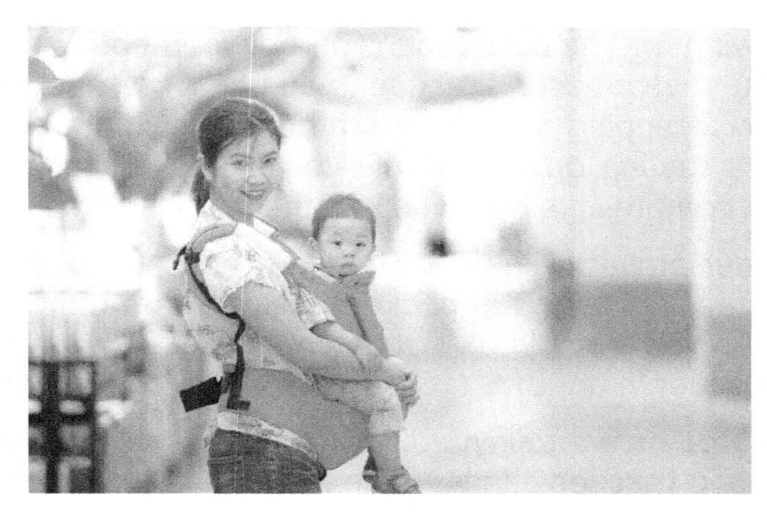

Image 27.

Action

It is crucial to **verify environmental safety**. Because you are inside and not in any type of danger, you know the scene is safe. Therefore, you **begin the initial assessment** by moving the infant's heel and shouting to determine responsiveness. You shout, but the infant does not respond in any way. You also quickly scan the victim's body for any other obvious injury, but you see nothing abnormal. No response from the infant indicates unresponsiveness and warrants **contacting the emergency response system**. As you yell for help, a bystander approaches the scene and states he is a nurse and can help. Another bystander begins to call 9-1-1 and runs to retrieve emergency equipment.

You place two fingers on the infant's inner upper arm to determine the presence of a brachial pulse. This is **completed in 10 seconds** while scanning the victim's chest for inspiration or expiration. Assessment reveals pulselessness and apnea.

You immediately **begin chest compressions**. You compress at a rate of 100-120 compressions per minute at a depth of at least 1.5

inches, allowing for chest re-expansion between each compression. Because you have a second rescuer, you utilize the encircling hands technique by wrapping your hands around the infant so that your fingertips are resting on the infant's lower back. Then, using both thumbs, you compress in the middle of the infant's chest.

A bystander arrives with an AED and a pocket mask. Therefore, the second rescuer uses the pocket mask to **administer 2 rescue breaths** after you complete 15 compressions. This is the correct ratio for 2-rescuer infant BLS (15 compressions for every 2 breaths).

After the breaths are delivered, you continue giving compressions and the second rescuer attaches the AED pads to the infant's bare chest and back. The bystander turns the device on, and the AED begins analyzing the infant's heart rhythm. You take your hands off the infant for heart rhythm analysis. The AED determines the infant does have a shockable heart rhythm. So, you continue chest compressions while the AED charges. When the AED is charged and ready to deliver a shock, you take your hands off the infant and the second rescuer ensures everyone is clear of the infant. The second rescuer provides a shock and then you switch roles. The second rescuer is now providing compressions while you administer breaths via the pocket mask. This is completed at a rate of 15 compressions for every 2 breaths.

After two minutes of CPR, the AED begins to analyze the infant's heart rhythm again. The second rescuer ceases compressions during heart rhythm analysis. This time, the infant's heart rhythm is deemed unshockable and you notice the infant start to wiggle his fingers and toes. You palpate and feel a weak, but present, brachial pulse. You both provide supportive care until the emergency response team arrives.

UNIT 4:
AIRWAY MANAGEMENT

Let's review and summarize what we have learned so far regarding airway management for adult, pediatric, and infant BLS victims. Then, we will discuss specialized topics such as advanced airways and rescue breathing.

CHAPTER 17:
REVIEW

Airway Maneuvers

Head tilt–chin lift

- Appropriate technique for adult, child, or infant victim who is unresponsive and needs an open airway.
- Only appropriate if the victim does not have a potential neck or head injury.
- After placing one hand on the victim's forehead, apply pressure to tilt the victim's head toward the ground. Next, take your other hand and position your fingers underneath the victim's chin. Lastly, pull the chin upward to open the airway and shift the tongue out of the way (AHA, 2016).
- Avoid pressing into the soft tissue at the anterior of the neck (AHA, 2016). This can create further oxygenation issues and hamper obstruction relief attempts.
- In infants, tilting the head back too far may obstruct the airway because of their anatomical prematurity. It is critical to not tilt the head "beyond the neutral (sniffing) position" (AHA, 2016, p. 52). Following this guideline ensures airway patency and proper positioning for oxygen delivery.

Jaw thrust

- Appropriate technique for adult, child, or infant victim with a potential head or neck injury who is unresponsive and needs an open airway.
- If this maneuver does not open the airway, you can switch to the head tilt–chin lift if the airway is obstructed.
- This maneuver takes adequate strength and two hands to complete; therefore, one rescuer will perform the jaw

thrust while the other delivers the oxygen (AHA, 2016).
- Stand directly behind the victim's head and place your elbows on the area behind the victim's head so that your hands can comfortably reach the jaw area (AHA, 2016). Next, "Place your fingers under the angles of the victim's lower jaw and lift with both hands, displacing the jaw forward" (AHA, 2016, p. 22). This allows you to relieve an obstruction and open the airway.

Airway Devices

Pocket mask

- The pocket mask comes in different sizes to accommodate adult, child, and infant victims. Most pocket masks are equipped with a one-way valve that ensures fluid expelled from the victim is not directed toward the rescuer (AHA, 2016).
- To correctly place a pocket mask, kneel or stand to the side of the victim. The "pointy" end of the pocket mask fits over the victim's nose with the wide part below the mouth. The mask should be pressed firmly against the victim's face so that a seal is created.
- To create a seal, use the index finger and thumb on the hand that is closest to the top of the victim to form a "C" shape around the air inlet. Your fingers should create a seal that prevents air leakage around the nose.
- Use the thumb of your opposite hand to compress the lower portion of the face mask to the victim's face. Use the fingers from the same hand to open the airway by lifting the jaw and completing a head tilt–chin lift.
- Lower yourself to the pocket mask and breathe into the mask. It will take 1 second to deliver an effective breath.

- You will know if your oxygen delivery was effective if you see the victim's chest rise with each delivered breath (AHA, 2016).

Bag valve mask (BVM)

- BVMs comes in different sizes to accommodate adult, pediatric, and infant victims.
- This device can be used while attached to oxygen or without supplemental oxygen.
- To deliver breaths with the BVM, you must stand or kneel above the victim's head. Next, use the "EC" method to ensure a tight seal around the victim's nose and mouth.
- For single-rescuer BVM use, place the mask on the victim's face with the "pointy" end over the nose and the wider portion below the mouth. Pull the bag toward the side you will be compressing while ensuring the bag is perpendicular to the victim's body. Keep the bag level so that the air supply is not cut off. Form a "C" shape with your thumb and index finger and wrap them around the mask, keeping close to the edge of the mask. The middle, ring, and pinky fingers will form an "E" and lift the jaw upward. This mimics a head tilt–chin lift. While ensuring a tight seal with one hand, use the other hand to compress the bag. A slow, steady squeeze will deliver an effective breath. You will know if your oxygen delivery was effective if you see the victim's chest rise with each bag compression (AHA, 2016).
- For 2-rescuer BVM use, your partner uses both hands to ensure the mask is completely sealed to the victim's face while you compress the bag to deliver the breath, or vice versa. Your partner will stand above the victim's head and position the mask over the victim's face while you stand to the side. Using the aforementioned "EC" method, your

partner seals the mask to the victim's face on one side and then mirrors this technique on the other side. This ensures a complete, circumferential seal. You can now gently squeeze the bag to deliver a breath at a slow, steady rate.

Unavailable Airway Equipment

Mouth-to-mouth breathing for adults, children, or infants:

1. Perform a head tilt–chin lift.
2. Use your index finger and thumb to close the victim's nose (AHA, 2016).
3. Make a seal with your mouth and provide one breath until you see the victim's chest rise (AHA, 2016).

Mouth-to-mouth-to-nose breathing for infants:

1. Perform a head tilt–chin lift.
2. Create an airtight seal by positioning "your mouth over the infant's mouth and nose" and provide one breath until you see the victim's chest or abdomen rise (AHA, 2016).

Airway Ratios

Victim	Single-Rescuer	2-Rescuer
Adult	30 compressions, then 2 breaths	30 compressions, then 2 breaths
Child	30 compressions, then 2 breaths	15 compressions, then 2 breaths
Infant	30 compressions, then 2 breaths	15 compressions, then 2 breaths

CHAPTER 18:
RESCUE BREATHING

Rescue breathing has a singular goal: provide breaths for a victim who is not breathing. Victims who require rescue breathing have a pulse present, whereas victims who require CPR do not have a pulse and are not breathing. It is important to differentiate abnormal breathing from agonal gasps because agonal gasps accompany or signal impending cardiac arrest; furthermore, presence of agonal gasps should prompt you to begin CPR (AHA, 2016).

For adult victims who have a pulse but are not breathing on their own, use the following steps:

1. Kneel or stand beside the victim.
2. Open the airway and place the appropriate airway device on the victim (e.g., pocket mask). If a device is unavailable, mouth-to-mouth breaths may be administered at your discretion. If completing mouth-to-mouth breaths, ensure the nose is pinched closed.
3. "Give 1 breath every 5 to 6 seconds" at a rate of approximately 10 to 12 breaths per minute (AHA, 2016, p. 62).
4. The victim's chest should rise with each rescue breath.

For child or infant victims who have a pulse but are not breathing on their own, use the following steps:

1. Kneel or stand beside the victim. It is appropriate to hold an infant victim and provide rescue breaths.
2. Open the airway and place the appropriate airway device on the victim (e.g., pocket mask). If a device is unavailable, mouth-to-mouth or mouth-to-mouth-to-nose

breaths may be administered. If completing mouth-to-mouth breaths, ensure the nose is pinched closed.
3. "Give 1 breath every 3 to 5 seconds" at a rate of approximately 12 to 20 breaths per minute (AHA, 2016, p. 62).
4. The victim's chest should rise with each rescue breath.

A critical element that must be highlighted for child or infant rescue breathing is the addition of chest compressions when the heart rate drops below 60 beats per minute. The victim will likely display signs of poor perfusion (e.g., weak pulse, paleness, mottling, and cyanosis). These signs and bradycardia indicate impending cardiac arrest and warrant the start of chest compressions (AHA, 2016).

CHAPTER 19:
ADVANCED AIRWAY

Compression-to-breath ratios change when the victim has an advanced airway in place. For this reason, knowledge of these ratios is imperative for proper airway management. The purpose of an advanced airway is to maintain a patent, open airway because a victim cannot. The airway is placed into the victim's trachea by a rescuer who has specialized training (e.g., paramedic or provider). Common advanced airways include an endotracheal (ET) tube, laryngeal mask airway (LMA), King airway, and Combitube. See Image 28, which depicts a placed ET tube.

TRACHEAL INTUBATION

endotracheal tube

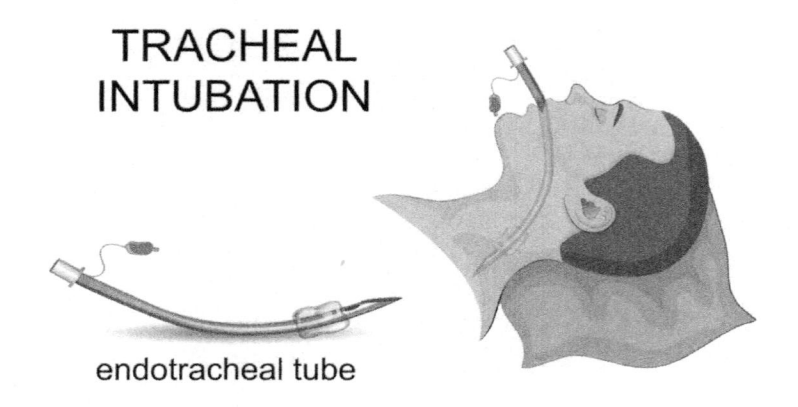

Image 28.

When an unconscious victim has an advanced airway in place, you should administer one breath through a BVM every 6 seconds. Therefore, the victim will receive 10 manual breaths every minute. This is the standard for adult, child, and infant victims.

One critical piece of BLS for a victim with an advanced airway in place is nonstop compressions. The compressor will no longer stop after 15 or 30 compressions (depending on the age of victim) to allow the other rescuer to deliver a breath. In other words, breaths and compressions can be given simultaneously with an advanced airway in place.

UNIT 5:
CHOKING

Choking is frightening to witness. A victim of choking often displays the "universal choking sign" by "clutching the throat with the thumb and fingers" (AHA, 2016, p. 71). See Image 29. An inability to speak will accompany severe choking. Therefore, you must direct the victim to answer through nodding if they're unable to respond when you ask, "Are you choking?" (AHA, 2016). Other signs that may accompany severe choking include cyanosis, inability to cough, and stridor (AHA, 2016).

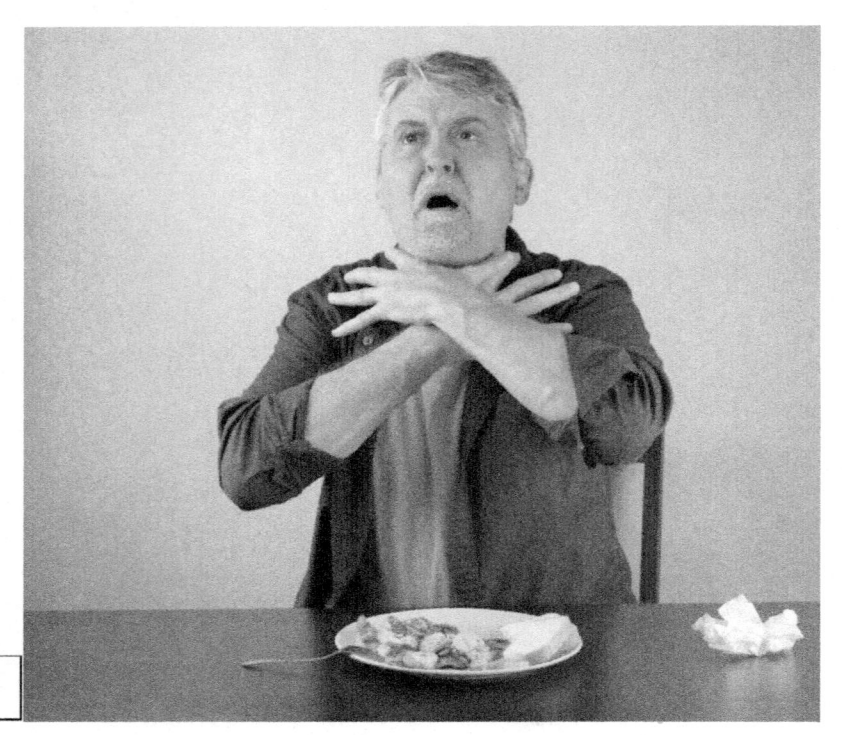

Image 29.

A bystander must be prepared to act quickly because an airway obstruction can result in death if left untreated. According to Duckett et al., the populations at highest risk for choking are infants, children, and older adults (2020). Common culprits of choking among children and infants include toys, food, and coins, whereas the cause of choking among older adults is primarily food (Duckett et al., 2020). The reality of the danger associated with choking is evidenced by the statistics. Duckett et al. report, "Choking is the fourth leading cause of unintentional death, the leading cause of infantile death, and the fourth leading cause of death among preschool children" (2020, para. 3).

These statistics are shocking and underscore the importance of choking relief measures. Furthermore, *everyone* should be knowledgeable on how to relieve choking. So, let's dive in and discuss how to relieve choking in adult, child, and infant victims.

CHAPTER 20:
RELIEF OF ADULT CHOKING

Choking relief in adults begins with positioning. When an adult victim is choking, stand behind the victim to adequately relieve airway obstruction. If you are much taller than the victim, you can kneel behind them instead. Next, encircle your arms around the victim and move closer to make contact. Without making direct contact with the victim, you won't be able to provide adequate resistance to relieve the obstruction.

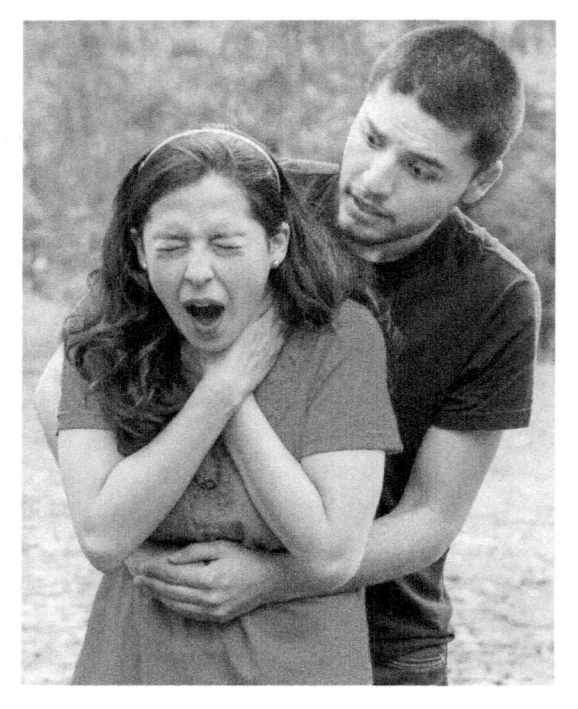

Image 30.

You should then take either hand and make a fist before positioning the fisted hand between the victim's belly button and breastbone. Your thumb should be flush against the victim. Using the other hand to cover the fisted hand, provide "a quick, forceful upward thrust" (AHA, 2016). Don't stop providing abdominal thrusts until the obstruction is relieved or upon victim collapse. This act of removing an airway obstruction is famously termed the *Heimlich maneuver* (AHA, 2016).

If the victim collapses and becomes unresponsive while performing the Heimlich maneuver, ensure the safety of the victim by gently placing the victim on the ground. You should then shout for help and call 9-1-1 (or direct a bystander to call 9-1-1). Without delay, begin providing chest compressions on a choking victim who is unresponsive. As a reminder, you should follow these guidelines:

- Kneel beside the victim.
- Place the heel of one hand in the middle of the victim's chest with the other hand interlocked.
- Keep your arms straight and compress with your body directly over the victim.
- Compress at least 2 inches.
- Complete 100-120 compressions per minute.
- Allow full chest expansion between compressions.
- Do not stop until AED arrival.

For an adult victim, compressions and breaths should be given at a rate of 30 compressions for every 2 breaths. Upon opening the airway through a maneuver such as the head tilt–chin lift, you should inspect the victim's mouth for the obstructing object. An easy-to-remember strategy for obstructing objects is "If you can see it, sweep it." In other words, if you see the object, carefully sweep it out with your fingers. If you cannot see the obstructing object, do not sweep because this could worsen the obstruction.

If the victim is pregnant or obese, don't perform abdominal thrusts between the belly button and the breastbone. Instead, your fisted hand should be placed on the victim's chest with the other hand on top. This technique provides appropriate choking relief for specialized cases.

You can confirm that choking relief measures were successful by observing the victim's chest moving upward when breaths are provided or if the obstruction itself is visualized in the victim's oral cavity (AHA, 2016).

Let's recap what we've learned about relief of adult choking by summarizing key points:

- Confirm whether the victim is choking. Signs of choking are the universal choking sign (see Image 29) or the victim being unable speak, cough, or clear the airway.
- Position yourself behind the victim so that your arms can easily reach the victim's abdomen.
- Encircle your arms around the victim and make a fist with one hand. Place the thumb of your fisted hand on the victim between the belly button and breastbone.
- Cover your fist with the other hand and provide upward thrusts until the obstruction is relieved or the victim collapses.
- If the victim becomes unresponsive, begin BLS protocol by calling 9-1-1 and beginning CPR.

CHAPTER 21:
RELIEF OF CHILD CHOKING

Relief of child choking closely mirrors relief of adult choking with one exception: positioning. While most adult rescuers will stand behind adult choking victims, almost all adult rescuers of child choking victims will kneel. You should be positioned behind the child so that your arms can comfortably reach the victim's abdomen (see Image 31).

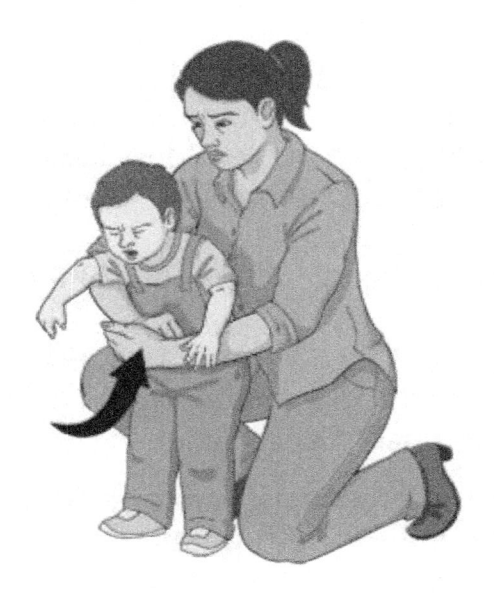

Image 31.

After getting into position, encircle your arms around the victim and move closer to make contact. Without making direct contact with the victim, you will not be able to provide adequate resistance to relieve the obstruction.

You should then take either hand and make a fist before positioning the fisted hand between the victim's belly button and breastbone. Your thumb should be flush against the victim. Using the other hand to cover the fisted hand, provide "a quick, forceful upward thrust" (AHA, 2016). Don't stop providing abdominal thrusts until the obstruction is relieved or upon victim collapse.

If the victim collapses and becomes unresponsive while performing the Heimlich maneuver, ensure the safety of the victim by gently placing the victim on the ground. You should then shout for help and call 9-1-1 (or direct a bystander to call 9-1-1). Without delay, begin providing chest compressions on a choking victim who is unresponsive. As a reminder, you should follow these guidelines:

- Kneel beside the victim.
- Place the heel of one hand in the middle of the victim's chest with the other hand interlocked.
- Keep your arms straight and compress with your body directly over the victim.
- Compress at least 2 inches (or 1/3 the AP diameter of the chest).
- Complete 100-120 compressions per minute.
- Allow full chest expansion between compressions.
- Do not stop until AED arrival.

In a child victim, compressions and breaths should be given at a rate of 30 compressions with 2 breaths if you are the only rescuer available. If there are 2 rescuers, the ratio changes to 15 compressions with 2 breaths.

Upon opening the airway through a maneuver such as the head tilt–chin lift, you should inspect the victim's mouth for the obstructing object. An easy-to-remember strategy for obstructing objects is "If you can see it, sweep it." In other words, if you see the object, carefully sweep it out with your fingers. If you cannot see the obstructing object, do not sweep because this could worsen the obstruction.

You can confirm that choking relief measures were successful by observing the victim's chest moving upward when breaths are provided or if the obstruction itself is visualized in the victim's oral cavity (AHA, 2016).

Let's recap what we've learned about relief of child choking by summarizing key points:

- Confirm whether the victim is choking. Signs of choking are the universal choking sign (see Image 29) or the victim being unable to speak, cough, or clear the airway.
- Position yourself behind the victim so that your arms can easily reach the victim's abdomen. Most adults will kneel behind child choking victims.
- Encircle your arms around the victim and make a fist with one hand. Place the thumb of the fisted hand on the victim between the belly button and breastbone.
- Cover your fist with the other hand and provide upward thrusts until the obstruction is relieved or the victim collapses.
- If the victim becomes unresponsive, begin BLS protocol by calling 9-1-1 and beginning CPR.

CHAPTER 22:
RELIEF OF INFANT CHOKING

Relief of infant choking is a completely different technique from the one used to relieve choking in adults and children. Let's explore these different choking relief measures in detail so that you can be prepared to intervene when necessary.

First, you must confirm whether the infant is choking by assessing the infant's level of consciousness. Determination can be made based on the infant's ability to make a noise, cough, or breathe while remaining conscious. Lack of noise, coughing, or breathing while conscious indicates airway obstruction.

As with all choking relief measures, you must position yourself properly. With an infant, you will hold the infant while sitting. The infant's head *must* be positioned below the rest of their body to promote obstruction relief via gravity. Failing to position the infant's head below the body hampers choking relief attempts.

One major difference between infant choking relief and adult/child choking relief is the elimination of abdominal thrusts. Abdominal thrusts are not used for infants because of anatomical differences and the potential to cause injury. Therefore, you will perform a series of "back slaps and chest thrusts" (AHA, 2016, p. 74).

Let's discuss the steps in the correct sequence of action after confirming the infant is choking:

1. Position the infant so that their head is facing away from you and below the rest of their body. Allow the infant to rest on your lower arm while holding the infant's head with your hand on the same arm. Avoid compressing the soft tissue of the throat, which can block the infant's airway further (see Image 32).
2. Place the arm with the infant against your leg for support.

3. Use your other hand to deliver 5 back slaps between the infant's shoulder blades. The back slaps should be given with an open-faced palm while using the heel of the hand.
4. Safely flip the infant over and complete 5 chest compressions using two fingers between the nipple line. During chest compressions, the infant's head should remain below the rest of their body.
5. Continue cycles of 5 back slaps followed by 5 chest compressions until the obstructing object becomes dislodged and/or visible or the infant loses consciousness.

If the infant becomes unresponsive while performing back slaps and chest compressions, place the victim on the ground or hard surface. You should then shout for help and call 9-1-1 (or direct a bystander to call 9-1-1). Without delay, you should begin providing CPR on a choking victim who is unresponsive. As a reminder, a rescuer providing chest compressions should follow these guidelines:

- For single-rescuer infant BLS chest compressions, compress in the middle of the infant's chest on the lower part of the breastbone.
- For 2-rescuer infant BLS chest compressions, wrap their hands around the infant so that the fingertips are resting on the infant's lower back. Then, using both thumbs, compress in the middle of the infant's chest.
- Complete 100-120 compressions per minute.
- Compress at least 1.5 inches (or 1/3 the AP diameter of the chest).
- Allow full chest expansion between compressions.

For an infant victim, compressions and breaths should be given at a rate of 30 compressions with 2 breaths if you are the only rescuer available. If there are 2 rescuers, the ratio changes to 15 compressions with 2 breaths.

Upon opening the airway through a maneuver such as the head tilt–chin lift, you should inspect the victim's mouth for the obstructing object. An easy-to-remember strategy for obstructing objects is "If you can see it, sweep it." In other words, if you see the object, carefully sweep it out with your fingers. If you cannot see the obstructing object, do not sweep because this could worsen the obstruction.

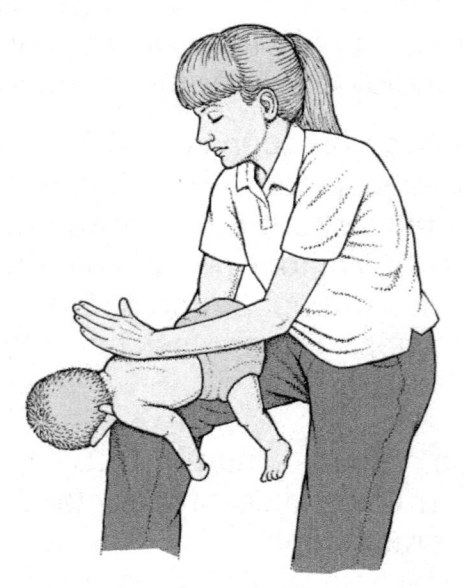

Image 32.

UNIT 6:
ALTERNATE TOPICS

The dynamics of BLS extend to other types of emergencies not caused by cardiac arrest. For example, opioid-induced emergencies are precipitated by the use or consumption of large doses of opioid medications. High concentrations of opioid medications trigger a chain of events that can ultimately lead to death if left untreated. These events include "central nervous system and respiratory depression that can cause respiratory and cardiac arrest" (AHA, 2016, p. 67). Within the United States, opioid overdose is considered an epidemic; the death toll caused by opioid misuse is 128 individuals daily (Centers for Disease Control and Prevention [CDC], 2020). The prevalence of this problem indicates bystanders must be prepared to act. Resuscitative efforts for individuals experiencing opioid overdose differ slightly from efforts for those who are experiencing other medical emergencies. For this reason, we will discuss management of opioid-induced emergencies separately.

One critical facet of BLS that is often overlooked is team synchrony. Without a smooth, functioning team, BLS efforts can be disjointed. The individual efforts of every rescuer must be communicated and acknowledged. As we discuss these last two topics of BLS, recall previous scenarios and consider different approaches to treatment if the precipitating event stemmed from opioid misuse. Also, consider the impact of effective teamwork and how the patient's survival ultimately relies on rescuers' collective efforts.

CHAPTER 23:
MANAGEMENT OF OPIOID-INDUCED EMERGENCY

An opioid is a type of medication that acts on the opioid receptors in the body and produces pain relief (National Institutes of Health, n.d.). Opioids can be prescribed for individuals who suffer from chronic or acute pain. Examples of these medications include oxycodone, hydrocodone, codeine, and morphine (NIH, n.d.). Some individuals misuse prescription opioids and non-prescription opioids, such as heroin and fentanyl.

According to the National Institute of Health (2017), continual use of opioids can induce tolerance (the individual requiring a larger dose to receive the same effects) and dependence (without continued usage, the individual experiences physical illness due to withdrawal). Long-term consequences of tolerance include misuse, addiction, and overdose. Therefore, careful monitoring by the provider and caution must be considered when managing acute and chronic pain with prescription opioids.

The effect of opioids can be counteracted by another medication: naloxone (AHA, 2016). In other words, this antidote can quickly "reverse the effects of respiratory depression caused by opioids" (AHA, 2016, p. 67). This medication has a short half-life, or the time it takes for a medication concentration to be reduced by half; therefore, multiple doses are often required during opioid overdoses. According to the AHA, naloxone is administered into the muscle (intramuscular), into the vein (intravascular), or through the nares (intranasal). Since we have covered the basics of opioids and their reversal agent, let's discover how to treat an individual who is experiencing an opioid overdose.

1. Upon approaching a victim who may be experiencing an opioid overdose, it is imperative that you ensure environmental safety. For example, you may need to maneuver or position around unsafe drug paraphernalia. Ensuring victim and rescuer environmental safety can be completed alongside observation for evidence of opioid use. This could include questioning others present at the scene, noticing drug paraphernalia, or seeing injection site marks on the victim (AHA, 2016).
2. Complete an initial assessment by evaluating the victim's responsiveness, shaking the victim's shoulder, and shouting to awaken the victim. You can shout, "Can you open your eyes?"
3. Contact the emergency response system by calling 9-1-1 or instructing a bystander to alert emergency personnel.
4. Complete a 10-second check by assessing for the presence of a pulse and breathing. For adult and child victims, you should palpate the carotid artery. For infant victims, palpate the brachial artery (inner upper arm).
5. If the victim has a palpable pulse, abnormal breathing, and a probable opioid overdose, provide rescue breaths and "administer naloxone per local protocols and monitor for response" (AHA, 2016, p. 69). Rescue breathing should continue until emergency personnel arrive and assume care. If the victim loses consciousness and becomes unresponsive, incorporate chest compressions and breaths.
6. If the victim is breathing abnormally and does not have a palpable pulse, provide chest compressions, breaths, and use the AED to perform immediate defibrillation if indicated. In addition, a probable opioid overdose warrants the administration of naloxone (AHA, 2016).

As a reminder, *adult* rescue breathing should include the following steps:

1. Kneel or stand beside the victim.
2. Open the airway and place the appropriate airway device on the victim (e.g., pocket mask). If a device is unavailable, mouth-to-mouth breaths may be administered at your discretion. If completing mouth-to-mouth breaths, ensure the nose is pinched closed.
3. "Give 1 breath every 5 to 6 seconds" at a rate of approximately 10 to 12 breaths per minute (AHA, 2016, p. 62).
4. The victim's chest should rise with each rescue breath.

Rescue breathing for *child or infant* victims should include the following steps:

1. Kneel or stand beside the victim. It is appropriate to hold an infant victim and provide rescue breaths.
2. Open the airway and place the appropriate airway device on the victim (e.g., pocket mask). If a device is unavailable, mouth-to-mouth breaths (or mouth-to-mouth-to-nose breaths for infants) may be administered. If completing mouth-to-mouth breaths, ensure the nose is pinched closed. Providing breaths for child and infant victims is imperative because they have a smaller blood oxygen reservoir than adult victims.
3. "Give 1 breath every 5 to 6 seconds (about 10 to 12 breaths per minute)" (AHA, 2016, p. 62).
4. The victim's chest should rise with each rescue breath.

A critical element that must be highlighted for child or infant rescue breathing is the addition of chest compressions when the heart rate drops below 60 beats per minute. The victim will likely display signs of poor perfusion (e.g., weak pulse, paleness, mottling, and cyanosis).

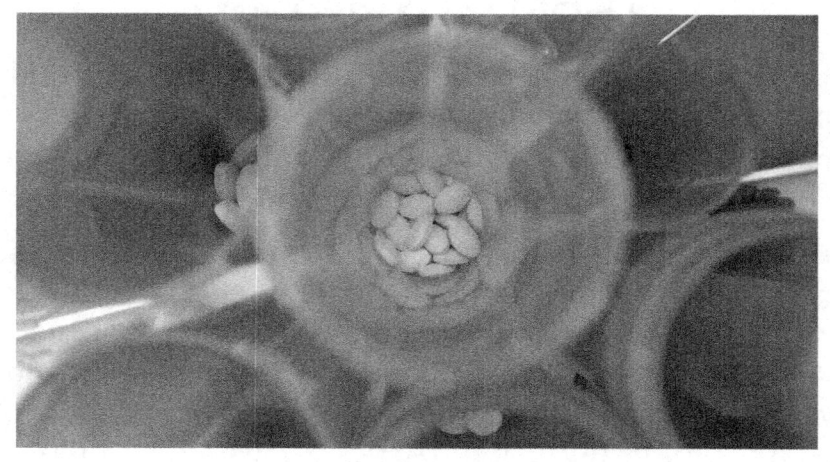

Image 33.

CHAPTER 24:
TEAM SYNCHRONY

In emergency situations, emotions are heightened, and panic is easily ignited. Patient survival largely depends on team efficiency; therefore, it is imperative for you and other rescuers to communicate with one another while remaining focused and calm.

Before we discuss the different roles of an effective team, let's identify one of the most impactful aspects of effective BLS teamwork —chest compressions. Continual, effective compressions must be counted and monitored. In addition, you must relieve one another every two minutes so that compression depth and quality remain adequate for organ perfusion (AHA, 2016). It is helpful for the compressors to count out loud, monitor each other's compressions, and communicate necessary modifications (e.g., "You are compressing too fast"). Without implementing these strategies, effective teamwork is compromised, and the victim suffers.

According to the AHA, a properly functioning BLS team requires six rescuers (2016). These rescuers will fulfill the following roles:

1. BLS lead: Delegate rescuer positions. Display calmness and sound judgement on critical decisions. Promote effective communication.
2. Airway management: Open the victim's airway and administer breaths.
3. Chest compressions: Provide continual chest compressions and pause when AED is analyzing or providing a shock. Compressions are also paused when breaths are given (unless victim has advanced airway).
4. AED use: Place electrodes/pads on the victim. Manage AED machine, including analyzing, charging, and providing shock. Switch positions with rescuer completing

chest compressions every two minutes to prevent compression fatigue.
5. Medication administration: Provide medications as per BLS Lead decisions.
6. Record events and monitor time: Provide summary of interventions and medications to BLS Lead. Documents events and medication administration.

As mentioned before, communication is imperative during BLS efforts. To expand upon this point, there is a specific type of communication that optimizes understanding and clarity. This is called *closed-loop communication*, and it must be used in these high intensity scenarios (AHA, 2016). This type of communication may seem over the top, but it decreases the risk for error and enhances patient outcomes. According to the AHA, each rescuer must make eye contact when communicating a point or giving an order (2016). Then, the rescuer receiving the message must confirm the communication. For example, the BLS Lead may tell the rescuer operating the AED to increase the energy level to 200 joules. After receiving the message, the AED operator must state back, "I am increasing the energy level to 200 joules."

After BLS efforts are rendered, the BLS Lead should gather the team to discuss the events that transpired. This is referred to as a *debriefing* (AHA, 2016). This invaluable time allows members to verbalize emotions, identify areas for improvement, and discuss positives (AHA, 2016). It is an important aspect of BLS that should be emphasized by all teams. It has been found that debriefings "improve patient survival after cardiac arrest" (AHA, 2016, p. 44). Let's be advocates of this crucial discussion for the sake of patient survival.

Printed in Great Britain
by Amazon